CARDIOLOGY

Management of Cardiac Arrest

Usually occurs in the context of acute myocardial infarction, but also with hypoxia, anaesthesia, surgery, shock, electrocution, drowning, hypothermia, biochemical abnormalities, drugs (digoxin, adrenaline), anaphylaxis, etc.

1. Establish the diagnosis – absent pulses, apnoea, unconsciousness.

2. Note the time.

3. A blow to the praecordium is occasionally successful in restoring normal rhythm.

4. Give an immediate DC shock with 400 J if a defibrillator is available. Do not delay defibrillation for lack of an ECG monitor as ventricular fibrillation is the commonest arrhythmia. Newer defibrillators may record the ECG via their paddles.

5. Begin external cardiac massage at about 60 compressions/min. Check efficiency at the femoral pulses. The patient must be on a hard surface, the floor if necessary.

6. Artificial respiration. First remove dentures and clear the airway. Use mouth to mouth ventilation if there is no equipment to hand, but use Brook airway/Ambu bag/endotracheal tube etc. if available. Ventilate with 100% oxygen. There is no reason for cardiac massage and ventilation to alternate; indeed, they are more efficient if simultaneous.

7. Establish an intravenous line. Give 8.4% bicarbonate, 1 ml/kg body weight; repeat every 10 min.

8. ECG monitor lead. Check the rhythm.
    (a) If VT or VF – 400 J DC shock. Repeat if necessary. If unsuccessful, give lignocaine 100 mg i.v. and repeat DC shock. If still unsuccessful with VF, give adrenaline 10 ml of 1 in 10,000 or 1 ml of 1 in 1000 i.v. and calcium chloride or gluconate 10 ml of 10% solution i.v. Repeat DC shock after further cardiac massage.
    (b) If asystole
        – adrenaline 1 ml of 1 in 1000 solution i.v.
        – calcium chloride or gluconate 10 ml of 10% solution i.v.
        – continue cardiac massage and ventilation.
        – repeat adrenaline and calcium after 5–10 min if required.
    (c) If fairly "normal" rhythm and no cardiac output, then a mechanical catastrophe is likely, e.g. ruptured ventricle, massive pulmonary embolism, tamponade. Try adrenaline, calcium and further massage.
9. Once stable
    (a) If the cause was VT or VF give lignocaine 100 mg i.v. over 2 min and then put up a lignocaine infusion at 4 mg/min for 30 min, then 3 mg/min for 30 min, then 2 mg/min.
    (b) Check arterial gases and serum potassium.
    (c) If the rhythm and output are restored but the patient does not breathe and the cause of the arrest is not clear, give naloxone 400–800 μg i.v. Repeat after 3–4 min if required.
    (d) If massive pulmonary embolism seems likely give heparin 15,000 units i.v.
    (e) Continue oxygen by mask.
    (f) Arrange a chest X-ray to look for pneumothorax, fractured ribs etc.

NOTE

1. In asystole or profound bradycardia, consider emergency pacing.
2. If tamponade is likely, immediate thoracotomy should be performed. Attempts at needle aspiration are pointless.
3. If resuscitation is successful but delayed and acute brain injury seems likely, consider
    (a) artificial ventilation
    (b) i.v. dexamethasone 12 mg stat then 4 mg 6–hourly
    (c) 20% mannitol 2.5 ml/kg stat then 0.5 ml/kg/hour
    (d) frusemide 40–80 mg i.v.

4. If there is significant hypokalaemia begin correction with 10–20 mmol potassium chloride i.v. over 5–10 min.

5. Do not give calcium into i.v. line containing bicarbonate as this will cause precipitation.

6. Pupillary dilatation is sometimes an unreliable guide to progress or lack of it.

7. It is more difficult to hit the heart with an intracardiac injection than might be expected and the heart may be damaged. The needle usually enters the right ventricle and thus is not necessarily more effective than an i.v. injection.

8. The various steps are listed in order of their urgency but, obviously, if plenty of help is available then several steps can be performed simultaneously.

D.C. Cardioversion

This section deals with synchronised DC cardioversion – for emergency cardioversion see "Cardiac Arrest".

INDICATIONS.

Most effective against
- ventricular tachycardia
- paroxysmal SVT
- atrial fibrillation
- atrial flutter
  especially if associated with haemodynamic embarrassment.
In AF consider cardioversion if
- of recent onset
- there is no identifiable underlying cause
- post-operative
- underlying thyrotoxicosis has been treated.
Usually ineffective if AF
- is secondary to mitral valve disease
- is associated with poor left ventricular function
- is longstanding (over 6 months)
- has relapsed after previous cardioversion.
Avoid cardioversion in
- sick sinus syndrome
- digoxin toxicity
- AF with complete heart block.

PRECAUTIONS

Usually performed under brief general anaesthetic (eg. i.v. metho-hexitone) with an anaesthetist and full resusitation facilities.

If urgent or no anaesthetist available it may be performed with i.v. diazepam.

In elective cardioversion for AF it is best to stop digoxin for a few days beforehand.

Anticoagulation: if cardioversion is an elective procedure for AF or atrial flutter, arrange oral anticoagulation for 2–4 weeks before and 2–4 weeks afterwards.

METHOD

1. Monitor the ECG on an oscilloscope.

2. Use a defibrillator which can be "synchronised" with the QRS complex on the patient's ECG. See precise instructions with machine.

3. Use jelly pads to avoid burning the skin (rather than electrode jelly).

4. In AF, especially if on digoxin, begin with a low energy level such as 20 J.

5. In VT start with 50–100 J.

6. If unsuccessful, try a higher energy shock.

7. Position one paddle below the right clavicle, the other on the lateral left chest wall (if a posterior paddle is used, it should be placed just below the left scapula).

8. Watch the ECG immediately after the shock
   - transient nodal rhythm is not uncommon
   - transient complete heart block occasionally occurs
   - if VF occurs give an immediate desynchronised shock of 200–400 J
   - if there is a bradycardia, consider i.v. atropine
   - ventricular extrasystoles are not uncommon
   - if asystole is produced, procede to immediate resuscitation (with isoprenaline and emergency pacing if necessary).

Consider maintainance treatment such as oral disopyramide to hold sinus rhythm.

Acute Myocardial Infarction

PRESENTATION

Usually with pain (but may be "silent"); also with pulmonary oedema, shock, syncope, and embolic complications.

EXAMINATION

Take particular note of general condition, pulse rate and rhythm, blood pressure, signs of cardiac failure, presence of pulses and murmurs.

INITIAL MANAGEMENT

1. Admit to a coronary care unit if possible.

2. Monitor the ECG as serious arrhythmias are common in the early stages.

3. i.v. cannula (for drugs and use in cardiac arrest). Avoid i.m. injections as they may affect serum enzymes.

4. Analgesia: i.v. diamorphine 2.5 mg repeated as necessary. Give with an antiemetic (cyclizine 50 mg or prochlorperazine 12.5 mg i.v.)

5. Give oxygen (35% or more) and frusemide 40–80 mg i.v. if there are signs of failure.

INVESTIGATIONS

ECG – note the date, time and whether the patient was in pain on all recordings.
  – normal progression   (a) ST elevation is the earliest sign
                            (b) Q waves (may not appear)
                            (c) T wave inversion is usually later.
  – may show ST depression, smaller R waves, bundle branch block or no change.
  – record at least daily for 3–4 days.
Chest X-ray – look for signs of failure (distended upper lobe veins, Kerley "B" lines, pulmonary oedema etc.).
Cardiac enzymes – those usually measured are creatinine kinase (CK), aspartate transaminase (AST), hydroxybutarate dehydrogenase (HBD) or lactate dehydrogenase (LDH). The normal time course is shown in Fig.1. This may influence the choice of enzymes estimated depending on

how soon the patient is seen after the onset of symptoms. Also consider other causes of abnormal enzyme results (liver disease, haemolysis, i.m. injections, etc.). Measure daily for the first 3 or 4 days and later if there is any suggestion of re-infarction

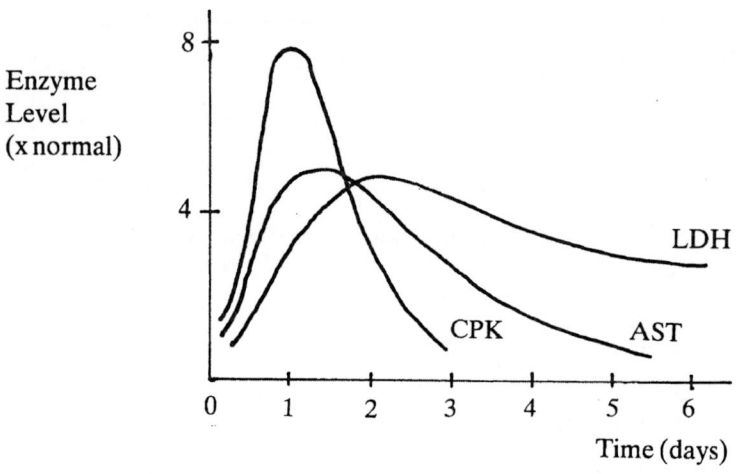

Figure 1
Pattern of serum enzyme elevation
following acute myocardial infarction.

Also check – WBC (often raised), haemoglobin, urea and electrolytes (potassium may need correction), blood glucose. Monitor the temperature chart as transient pyrexia is common.

Mobilisation – depends on the patient's age, size of infarction, complications and other diseases. The average is about 2 days in bed and 10 days in hospital; slower if heart failure, angina or re-infarction occur.

Rehabilitation – early exercise testing, before discharge with a modified protocol, is becoming widely used and has important prognostic significance. Most patients will be off work until the first review appointment at 4–6 weeks and the course thereafter depends on age, infarct size, occupation, motivation etc.

Reassurance – explain and reassure at every stage. Many hospitals distribute explanatory leaflets for patients to read.

Anticoagulation – in the acute phase, prevents DVT and pulmonary embolism but has not been shown to influence the course of infarction. A common compromise is sub-cutaneous heparin 5000 units b.d.

Risk factors – ban smoking, treat hypertension, and encourage weight loss. In the acute phase serum lipids are artificially low and difficult to interpret. Check the lipid profile at outpatient review in younger patients.

At the follow up clinic check – does the patient have angina?
　　　　　　　　　　　　　　 – are there any signs of failure?
　　　　　　　　　　　　　　 – measure the blood pressure
　　　　　　　　　　　　　　 – consider fasting lipid profile.

COMPLICATIONS

Arrhythmias

1.　Sinus bradycardia (see Fig. 2a)
　　　　–common, especially in inferior infarction.
　　　　–treat with atropine 0.6 mg i.v. if rate below 40/min or hypotensive. Repeat as necessary.

2.　Sinus tachycardia (see Fig. 2b)
　　　　–usually reflects pain, anxiety, heart failure or shock. Treat the underlying problem.

3.　Nodal or supra-ventricular tachycardia (see Fig. 2c)
　　　　–try carotid sinus massage first. Use cardioversion if shocked, otherwise practolol 10–20 mg i.v. slowly, repeated after 15 min if necessary or verapamil 1 mg/min i.v. up to 10 mg, but not both drugs, because there is a risk of asystole.

4.　Atrial flutter and fibrillation (see Figs. 2d & 2e)
　　　　–often transient. Both arrhythmias respond well to DC cardioversion if haemodynamic disturbance is present. Otherwise give verapamil as above or deslanoside 800–1200 μg i.v. (cardiac glycosides are better avoided in acute infarction if possible, but controlling the ventricular rate may be more important).

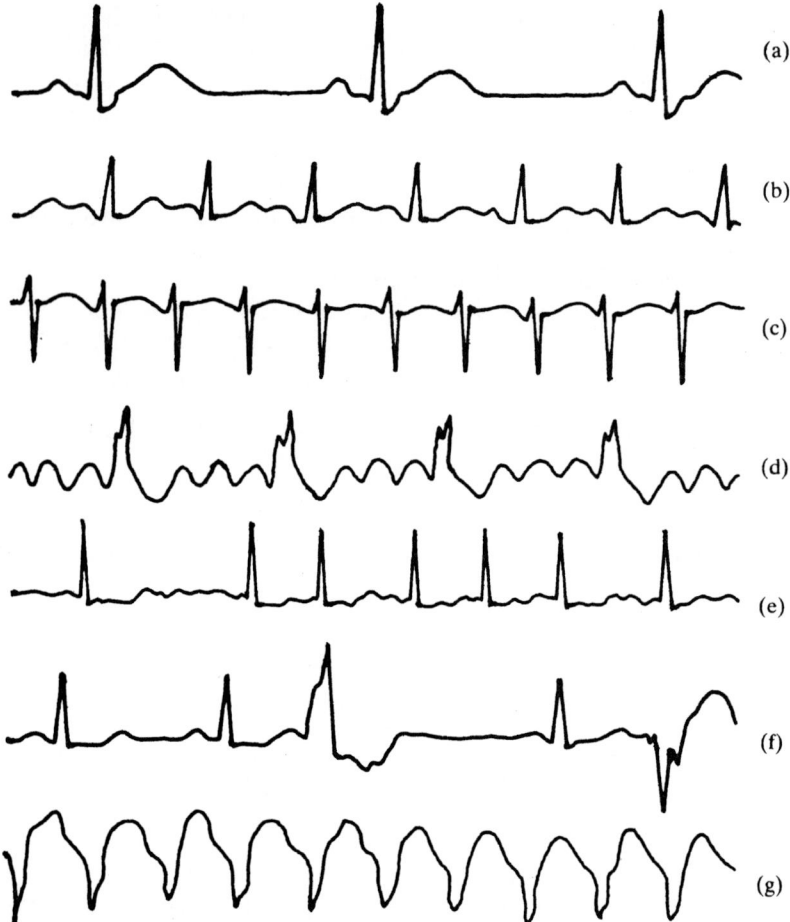

Figure 2

(a) Sinus bradycardia — sinus rhythm with rate below 60/min;

(b) Sinus tachycardia — sinus rhythm with rate above 100/min;

(c) Supra-ventricular tachycardia — QRS complexes usually narrow;

(d) Atrial flutter — conduction is usually 2:1 or 4:1

(e) Atrial fibrillation — irregular QRS complexes with no P waves;

(f) Ventricular ectopics — broad premature complexes, usually with a compensatory pause

(g) Ventricular tachycardia — broad complexes, usually 150-250/min and more or less regular: look for independent P waves

5. Atrial ectopics
    – common, and do not require treatment. May precede atrial fibrillation.

6. Ventricular ectopics (see Fig. 2f)
    – very common. Evidence that their suppression is beneficial is now less convincing. "R on T" ectopics are the most ominous. If the sinus rate is below 60, give atropine, if above 110 give practolol. Otherwise use lignocaine as below.

7. Ventricular tachycardia (see Fig. 2g)
    – if shock or syncope use immediate DC cardioversion. Otherwise give lignocaine 50–150 mg i.v. followed by an infusion of 4 mg/min, reducing to 2 mg/min. If ineffective, use disopyramide 2 mg/kg i.v. over 5 min to a maximum of 150 mg and up to 300 mg in the first hour; or mexiletine 150–250 mg i.v. over 5 min, and, failing that, or with a recurrence, a combination of drugs may be needed. Overdrive pacing may also help if drugs fail (see "Temporary Pacing").

8. Ventricular fibrillation (see Fig. 3a)
    – immediate defibrillation, 200–400 J
    See "Cardiac Arrest"

9. Accelerated idioventricular rhythm (AIR) (see Fig. 3b)
    – common, and rarely needs treatment. Responds to i.v. atropine.

10. First degree heart block (see Fig. 3c)
    – common especially in inferior infarction. Do not treat. Watch with repeat ECGs. Avoid digoxin.

11. Second degree heart block
    (a) Wenckebach (see Fig. 3d)
        – common in inferior infarction and usually benign. If necessary give i.v. atropine.
    (b) Mobitz II (see Fig. 3e)
        – may progress to complete block. Usually an indication for temporary pacing. Differentiate from non-conducted atrial ectopics.
    (c) 2 to 1 block (see Fig. 3f)
        – may be Wenckebach (in 90%) or Mobitz II (more

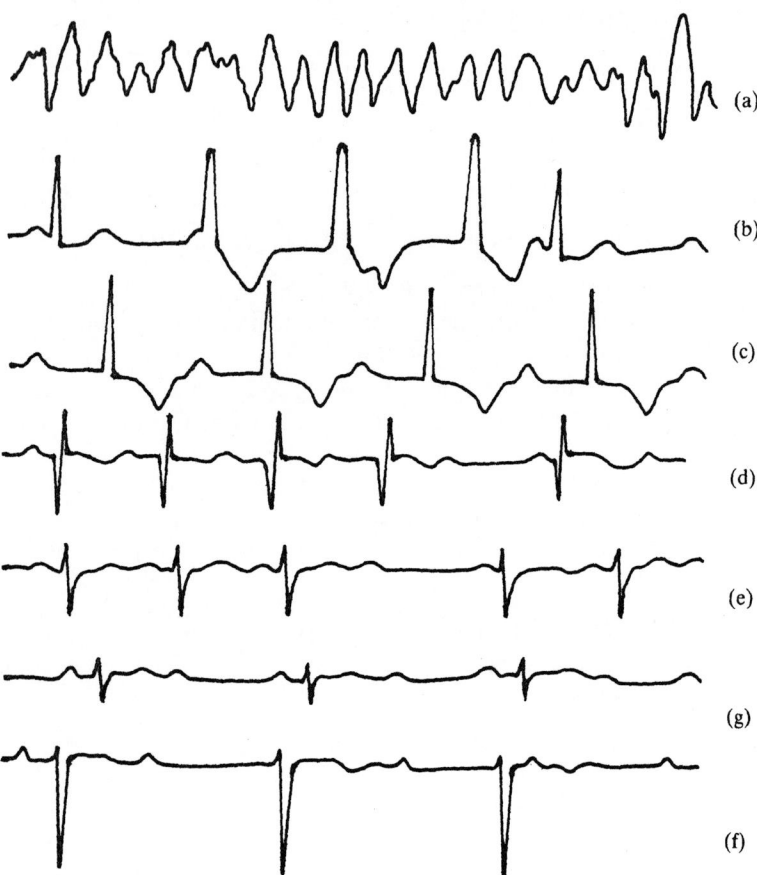

Figure 3
(a) Ventricular fibrillation—unco-ordinated electrical activity.
(b) Accelerated idio-ventricular rhythm—broad QRS complexes between 60 and 100/min and faster than the sinus rate;
(c) First degree heart block—PR interval greater than 0.22 second;
(d) Wenckebach second degree block—increasing PR interval with dropped QRS.
(e) Mobitz II second degree block—constant PR interval with dropped QRS;
(f) 2:1 second degree block—alternate P waves are conducted;
(g) Complete heart block—unrelated P waves and QRS complexes. The QRS is narrow in this example

likely if BBB is present). Try atropine 0.6 mg i.v. or temporary pacing if the bradycardia produces hypotension.

12. Complete heart block (CHB)(see Fig. 3g)

CHB with a narrow QRS in inferior MI is common. Treat with atropine if there is a significant bradycardia. Isoprenaline infusion may be used until temporary pacing can be arranged if there is haemodynamic embarassment.

CHB with broad QRS in anterior MI - ominous, often implying extensive infarction. Insert a temporary pacemaker. May take up to 3 weeks to resolve and occasionally a permanent pacemaker is needed.

13. Indications for temporary pacing in acute infarction.

(a) almost always in
- CHB with anterior infarction
- Mobitz II second degree block
- intermittent ventricular standstill.

(b) often advised in
- new RBBB and left posterior hemiblock
- new RBBB and left anterior hemiblock (LAHB) with long PR interval.

(c) occasionally in
- CHB with inferior infarction
- new LBBB
- new RBBB and LAHB
- any symptomatic bradycardia
- resistant VT (overdrive pacing).

Failure

- present if there are basal crepitations, third heart sound, congestion on chest X-ray.
- treat with frusemide 40 mg , repeat if necessary.
- maintenance treatment is not always needed and a thiazide may be sufficient. If not, use frusemide and then as the next step add isosorbide. Potassium replacement is necessary.
- see also "Pulmonary Oedema"

Shock

- see under "Cardiogenic Shock"

Pericarditis
- common; the friction rub is often transient and may be absent. Usually responds to indomethacin 25 mg t.d.s.

Onset of Murmur
- a quiet systolic murmur is common. No treatment is necessary if the patient is haemodynamically stable.
- a loud pansystolic murmur with a third heart sound, a thrill, clinical deterioration and often shock or pulmonary oedema: the differential diagnosis is between a ruptured ventricular septum and acute mitral regurgitation. Refer for investigation.

LATER PROBLEMS

1. Dressler's syndrome
   - uncommon. Presents at 2–6 weeks with pain, failure, pleural and pericardial effusions, fatigue, fever, pericardial rub.
   - check temperature, ESR, ECG, cardiac enzymes, anticardiac antibodies.
   - treat with an analgesic and consider a course of prednisolone if severe.

2. Left ventricular aneurysm
   - suggested by persisting failure, arrhythmias, emboli, paradoxical apex beat.
   - chest X-ray may show a "boot-shaped" heart.
   - ECG may show persisting ST elevation.
   - consider referral for investigation (the diagnosis can often be confirmed non-invasively with gated blood pool scanning or a 2D echocardiogram).

3. Emboli
   - from mural thrombus, see under "Systemic Emboli".

Cardiac Arrhythmias

Cardiac arrhythmias are considered in detail under "Acute Myocardial Infarction" but also occur in circumstances where the indications and recommendations for treatment may be different.

1. Paroxysmal supraventricular tachycardia (see Fig. 2c)
   - regular, usually above 150/min.

- distinguish from sinus tachycardia, AF, atrial flutter, VT.
- causes include ischaemia, Wolff-Parkinson-White and Lown-Ganong-Levine syndromes, and digoxin toxicity, but often none is found.

(a) if the patient is well and the attacks are self limiting, it may be sufficient to observe for a while.

(b) try carotid sinus massage.

(c) use DC cardioversion if there is haemodynamic embarassment.

(d) drugs – verapamil 5–10 mg i.v. slowly
    OR – practolol 5–20 mg i.v. slowly
    OR – disopyramide 2 mg/kg
    OR – digoxin (see "Digoxin")

If one drug fails another may be given later, but not verapamil **AND** practolol, and take care with disopyramide and verapamil.

(e) for long term prevention a beta-blocker or disopyramide is the drug of choice.

2. Atrial fibrillation (see Fig. 2e)
    - irregularly irregular with absent P waves.
    - seen in ischaemic, valvular, thyrotoxic and alcoholic heart disease, cardiomyopathy, ASD, pericarditis etc.
    - usually treated with digoxin (for doses see "Digoxin").
    - if not fully controlled add a beta-blocker or verapamil.
    - to prevent recurrence of paroxysmal AF try disopyramide or amiodarone or procainamide.

3. Atrial flutter (see Fig. 2d)
    - the ventricular rate is often almost exactly 150/min (i.e. 2:1 conduction) when untreated.
    - seen in ischaemia, cardiomyopathy, after cardiac surgery, etc.
    - responds well to DC shock or overdrive pacing.
    - treat with digoxin or beta-blocker or verapamil as above.
    - beware of disopyramide which may slow the flutter rate enough to allow 1:1 conduction and thereby increase the ventricular rate.

4. Sinus bradycardia (see Fig. 2a)
    - sinus rhythm below 60/min.
    - seen in normal people, athletes, sino-atrial disease, drug treatment (digoxin, beta blockade), myxoedema, raised

intracranial pressure etc.
 – rarely needs acute treatment but, if prolonged and symptomatic, permanent pacing is sometimes required.

5. Ventricular ectopics (see Fig. 2f)
    – very common but rarely require treatment.
    – apart from infarction they may be important in hypertrophic cardiomyopathy and in patients taking digoxin.

6. Ventricular tachycardia (see Fig. 2g)
    – by definition is a run of three or more ventricular ectopics.
    – with a broad-complex tachycardia it is sometimes difficult to distinguish between VT and SVT with aberration. The following may help:
    (a) look for independent P waves in VT and related P waves in SVT.
    (b) capture beats and fusion beats are seen in VT.
    (c) if there is a classical LBBB or RBBB pattern, SVT with aberration is more likely.
    (d) in lead V1 if R is taller than R', VT is likely.
    (e) if the QRS is predominantly upright in all chest leads, VT is more likely.
   – the main causes are ischaemic heart disease and digoxin toxicity. VT may be a cause of Stokes-Adams attacks in complete heart block.
   – in the acute situation, treatment is as detailed under "Acute Myocardial Infarction". If not related to an acute problem, oral suppressive treatment will be necessary:
           oral disopyramide 100–150 mg 6 or 8 hourly
           oral mexiletine 200–300 mg 8 hourly
           oral amiodarone 400 mg daily

Management of Acute Pulmonary Oedema

CLINICAL FEATURES

Increasing dyspnoea, orthopnoea, paroxysmal nocturnal dyspnoea, sweating cough and pink sputum and cardiac pain.

DIAGNOSIS

On history, chest auscultation and chest X-ray.

CAUSES

Myocardial infarction, hypertension, beta-blockers, valve disease (especially with the onset of uncontrolled AF), overtransfusion.

DIFFERENTIAL DIAGNOSIS

Asthma, acute – on – chronic bronchitis, pulmonary embolism, severe pneumonia, etc.

MANAGEMENT

1. Sit the patient up.

2. Give 40% oxygen by mask or nasal catheter (if the patient also has chronic chest disease, monitor blood gases).

3. Drugs
   - diamorphine 2.5 mg i.v. repeated as necessary (have naloxone available). Avoid in chronic lung disease or if the diagnosis is in doubt. It may be safer to give 1 mg at a time.
   - anti-emetic; cyclizine 50 mg or prochlorperazine 12.5 mg i.v. with the diamorphine.
   - frusemide 40–80 mg i.v.
   - aminophylline 250–500 mg i.v. slowly.
   - digoxin, if the patient is not on digoxin and there is no evidence of acute infarction (see "Digoxin").
   - vasodilators: glyceryl trinitrate, nitroprusside, isosorbide. Nitroprusside is first choice in hypertensive heart failure, although a mild elevation of blood pressure is common in pulmonary oedema.

4. Specific treatment of dysrhythmia. VT and uncontrolled AF may be best treated by cardioversion.

5. Venesection is best for overtransfusion.

6. Consider mechanical ventilation if no improvement.

7. A Swan-Ganz catheter may help in management, especially if vasodilators or ventilation are used.

8. Once the situation is stable, identify the cause. If none is obvious, consider rarer causes eg. myxoma, inhaled gases, etc.

9. In valve disease, if there is no improvement, consider referral for urgent investigation and operation.

10. Check Hb, albumin, urea and electrolytes, and cardiac enzymes.

11. Monitor improvement clinically and with fluid balance, daily weight and repeat chest X-ray.

12. Drain pleural effusion if large enough to be contributing to dyspnoea.

Management of Cardiogenic Shock

DEFINITION

A syndrome produced by pump failure and characterised by hypotension (systolic <80 mmHg), oliguria and peripheral vasoconstriction, often accompanied by pulmonary oedema.

CAUSES

- acute myocardial infarction
- acute mitral or aortic regurgitation
- acute ventricular septal defect
- cardiac tamponade

DIFFERENTIAL DIAGNOSIS

Includes haemorrhage, septicaemia, massive pulmonary embolism.

MANAGEMENT

1. Identify any treatable causes (e.g. acute VSD in infarction).

2. Before treatment, *THINK* - in view of the poor prognosis is aggressive treatment justified in this patient? Does age or other disease suggest it would be best to avoid invasive procedures with little hope of success?

3. Give oxygen by face mask or nasal cannulae.

4. Treat pain with diamorphine 2.5 mg i.v. as required.

5. Haemodynamic monitoring
   - Swan-Ganz catheter via subclavian vein to monitor pulmonary wedge pressure.
   - peripheral arterial line for BP and blood gases.
   - urinary catheter to measure hourly output.

6. If the wedge pressure is below 18–20 mmHg, raise to this level by infusion of normal saline (to provide preload for the left ventricle).

7. Commence low dose infusion of nitroprusside if BP allows, but watch BP carefully.

8. Begin dopamine infusion
   – at 2.5–5.0 μg/kg/min renal blood flow, cardiac output and contractility increase.
   – above 5–10 μg/kg/min, peripheral resistance and heart rate increase, thus increasing cardiac work.
   – watch for dysrhythmias.

9. Dobutamine infusion up to 10 μg/kg/min produces an increase in cardiac output while reducing LV filling pressure. There is less effect on rate and less irritability than with dopamine. It can be used in combination with dopamine and nitroprusside.

10. Intra-aortic balloon counterpulsation, if available, can improve and stabilise the situation, allowing time for investigation.

11. If there is no obvious cause, an echocardiogram must be done to exclude tamponade or left atrial myxoma.

Pericardial Tamponade

CAUSES

Trauma (may be non-penetrating), malignancy, uraemia, infection, aortic dissection, connective tissue diseases.

SYMPTOMS

Dyspnoea, fatigue, faintness, pain, collapse.

PHYSICAL SIGNS

Tachycardia, raised JVP, hypotension, pulsus paradoxus (more than 10 mmHg fall in systolic BP on inspiration), friction rub.

INVESTIGATIONS

Echocardiography – the investigation of choice if available.
Chest X-ray – may show cardiomegaly.

ECG – low voltage and T wave inversion (non specific).
Screening with a catheter in the right atrium or a right atrial angiogram are now rarely indicated but may help with the diagnosis if no other facilities are available.

PERICARDIAL ASPIRATION

Indications
  – hypotension, marked signs, deterioration, and to provide fluid for investigations.

Technique
  – the xiphisternal route is preferable.
  – use a lumbar puncture needle under local anaesthetic.
  – advance the needle to the left of the xiphisternum, cephalad at 45 degrees and aimed slightly to the left.
  – ECG monitoring via the needle is often advocated but may be difficult to use because of respiratory swing on the trace.
  – send fluid for Hb and PCV, protein, sugar, cytology, culture and Gram stain.
  – if a large volume is present a cannula may be used to facilitate aspiration and reduce the risk of damage to the heart.

Complications
  – include RV puncture, coronary artery or vein laceration and pneumothorax.
Refer for surgical drainage if
  – haemopericardium
  – malignant effusion
  – rapid recurrence.

Pericarditis and Pericardial Effusion

The causes of each are similar and the list of aetiologies suggests the necessary investigations.

CAUSES

  – viral, bacterial, tuberculous infection
  – myocardial infarction
  – malignant infiltration
  – congestive heart failure, uraemia, hypoalbuminaemia

– trauma, post-cardiotomy syndrome, post radiotherapy
– Dressler's syndrome, myxoedema, SLE.

INVESTIGATIONS

Chest X-ray – often normal. At least 250 ml of fluid are needed to produce enlargement of the cardiac shadow.

ECG – widespread ST elevation in awk pericarditis, classically concave upwards. T wave changes, low voltage, and electrical alternans are seen in pericardial effusion.

Echocardiogram – the best way to demonstrate an effusion.

Other investigations as suggested by the list of causes.

Pericardiocentesis is useful to establish the diagnosis in bacterial, tuberculous and malignant pericarditis.

MANAGEMENT

1. Analgesia.

2. Watch for signs of tamponade (see above).

3. Establish the cause as above.

4. Specific treatment depending on the cause.

Management of Chronic Stable Angina

HISTORY

Establish the diagnosis and its severity from the history. Distinguish from other causes of chest pain as far as possible. Also ask about past hypertension, myocardial infarction, risk factors (smoking, obesity, etc.) and diseases affecting the choice of treatment (asthma, peripheral vascular disease, etc.).

EXAMINATION

Measure BP, look for signs of heart failure and peripheral vascular disease.

Factors other than ischaemic heart disease may contribute to or cause angina (eg anaemia, aortic stenosis).

ECG – will be normal in over 50%.

Chest X-ray – normal unless heart failure or hypertension etc. are present.

FBC – if anaemia is present, its correction will often improve angina.

Lipids – check fasting profile in younger patients.

Exercise testing – very helpful but if negative does not exclude the diagnosis. Useful in assessing severity and response to treatment and in identifying those patients with severe disease.

Coronary arteriography – indicated in patients in whom medical treatment has failed, in those who may have severe disease, and when a job may be at risk (e.g. pilots, drivers).

MANAGEMENT

1. Explain the diagnosis and reassure the patient. Stress the good prognosis.

2. Correct any risk factors – hypertension, smoking, obesity etc.

3. Start glyceryl trinitrate. Explain its use, particularly as prophylaxis before exertion. It should be taken as often as needed.

4. The next stage is a beta-blocker if not contra-indicated (by asthma, cardiac failure, vascular disease). Use propranolol unless a cardio selective drug is indicated. Begin with 40 mg t.d.s. and increase as necessary. Change to another beta-blocker if minor side-effects are troublesome.

5. Add a long-acting nitrate, such as isosorbide dinitrate 10 mg t.d.s. Increase the dose if well tolerated.

6. Consider adding nifedepine, perhexiline, lidoflazine, or verapamil, especially in those in whom investigation and/or surgery is ruled out by age, past infarction, or other illnesses.

7. Consider coronary arteriography with a view to coronary bypass grafting. Except in the case of left main stem stenosis and triple vessel disease the decision is made on the basis of symptoms so there must be no doubt about the diagnosis and its severity before investigation. Arteriography is rarely indicated to confirm or exclude the diagnosis.

Management of Unstable Angina

DEFINITION

Includes patients with progressive angina of recent onset, those with rapidly worsening angina, and pain at rest.

ECG

Shows variable ST/T changes or may be normal if pain-free. ST depression and T wave inversion are not uncommon.
Prinzmetal angina produces ST segment elevation during pain.

MANAGEMENT

1. Bed rest.
2. Glyceryl trinitrate tablets as required. Topical GTN paste is often useful.
3. Diamorphine if no relief or for prolonged pain.
4. A beta-blocker, increasing the dose as necessary to produce a resting bradycardia.
5. Add isosorbide 10–20 mg q.d.s., increasing rapidly if pain persists. Can also be given by infusion.
6. Verapamil 40–80 mg or more t.d.s. and nifedepine 10–20 mg t.d.s. are further possibilities.
7. Heparin is sometimes advocated. So far there is no proof that it influences the incidence of infarction, but it will help to prevent DVT or pulmonary embolism.
8. Refer for coronary arteriography if the pain does not settle rapidly. The patient can often be stabilised on intra-aortic balloon pumping and this may be necessary before investigation.

Management of Hypertension

HISTORY

Most patients are asymptomatic.
Ask about
- complications such as angina, claudication, previous myocardial infarction or stroke
- contributory factors: family history, obesity, salt intake
- others risk factors: smoking, diabetes, diet
- medication.

EXAMINATION

Measure BP at rest, with the patient relaxed.
Assess target organ damage: fundi, LV hypertrophy, peripheral pulses.
Look for an underlying cause: femoral pulses, Cushingoid facies, renal masses, renal bruits.

INVESTIGATIONS

Chest X-ray – looking for cardiomegaly, rib notching, pulmonary congestion.
ECG – may show left ventricular hypertrophy.
Urine – stick testing and microscopy.
Serum urea, creatinine and electrolytes.
Investigation rarely reveals an underlying cause but may be indicated in younger patients or where the history, examination or simple tests suggest an underlying disease.
Renal artery stenosis – often a bruit present. IVP is suggestive in 70% of cases. Confirm with renal vein renin samples and renal arteriography.
Conn's syndrome – suggested by ↓K, ↑Na, and ↑ bicarbonate on biochemical screen if not on a diuretic. Confirm with plasma renin (low) and aldosterone (high).
Cushing's syndrome – typical clinical features, glycosuria, hypokalaemia. Further investigations include diurnal plasma cortisol levels, 24 hour urinary cortisol and low dose dexamethasone suppression test.
Phaeochromocytoma – history of anxiety, sweating, tremor and palpitation. The hypertension is often sustained. Check 24 hour urinary VMA excretion on several samples. Confirm with plasma catecholamines.
Coarctation of the aorta – suggested by delayed or absent femoral pulses, a systolic murmur, evidence of collateral vessels (especially around the scapulae) and by abnormal aortic knuckle and rib-notching on chest X-ray.

TREATMENT

1. Correct other risk factors.

2. Encourage weight loss and reduce salt intake.

3. Drugs
    (a) begin with a beta-blocker (eg. propranolol 40 mg b.d. or

atenolol 100 mg daily) in younger patients.

(b) use a thiazide diuretic (eg. bendrofluazide 5 mg daily) in older patients.

(c) combine beta-blocker and thiazide if control is not achieved after a few weeks.

(d) a vasodilator eg. prazosin or hydralazine is usually the next step in resistant cases.

(e) consider methyl dopa, labetalol, or debrisoquine if the above regime fails.

(f) newer drugs for resistant hypertension include minoxidil and captopril.

(g) remember that non-compliance is a common cause of treatment "failure".

The level of hypertension to treat and the degree of control to accept remain controversial. Treat, and aim for, lower pressures in younger patients. Use the above format as a guide only.

Accelerated Hypertension

Hypertension should be regarded as an emergency if any of the following is present:

1. diastolic pressure greater than 140 mmHg

2. pulmonary oedema

3. encephalopathy

4. renal failure

5. aortic dissection.

In the first instance do not reduce the blood pressure too quickly, or aim to reduce it below 150/100. Aortic dissection is an exception, where a systolic of 100–110 mmHg is preferable.

TREATMENT

1. Labetalol
   - mix 200 mg in 200 ml of dextrose-saline.
   - infuse 2 mg/min until a satisfactory response is obtained.
   - the usual dose needed is in the range 50–200 mg.
   - once controlled, transfer to oral treatment.

2. Nitroprusside
   - begin with 0.5–1.5 μg/kg/min.

- increase to 0.5–8 μg/kg/min depending on response.
- effective dose is usually in the range 50–400 μg/min.
- the maximum dose is 800 μg/min.
- treatment of choice in LVF or aortic dissection.
- avoid in patients with renal or hepatic failure.
- protect from light and avoid extravasation.
- monitor BP carefully.
- do not stop infusion suddenly.

3. Hydralazine
    - 20–40 mg i.v. slowly or by infusion.
    - may cause tachycardia and worsening of angina.

4. Propranolol and hydralazine orally will often produce a satisfactory response, even when hypertension is severe.

Dissecting Aneurysm of the Aorta

PRESENTATION

Pain (sudden, severe, tearing pain in the back, chest and abdomen), collapse, shock and stroke.

EXAMINATION

Measure the BP (often raised although the patient looks shocked).
Check all peripheral pulses.
Look for signs of peripheral ischaemia (stroke, paraplegia, silent abdomen, cold leg, etc).
Listen carefully for an aortic diastolic murmur.

INVESTIGATIONS

Chest X-ray
    - widening of the mediastinum is common but may take time to develop.
    - a small left pleural effusion may be present.
ECG
    - changes of left ventricular hypertrophy due to hypertension are often seen.
    - acute infarction changes may be present.

MANAGEMENT

1. Admit to intensive care unit if possible.

2. Relieve pain with i.v. diamorphine.

3. Establish venous and arterial lines.

4. If hypertensive, begin nitroprusside infusion (see under "Accelerated Hypertension").

5. Refer for emergency aortography. In general, surgical treatment is better for type I and II dissections (involving the ascending aorta) and medical, i.e. hypotensive, treatment for type III which are more distal. In time CAT scanning may be a rapid non-invasive technique to distinguish between them.

Note

Decisions about management and surgery will obviously be affected by the presence of stroke or other complications and the age and previous health of the patient.

Management of Congestive Cardiac Failure

DEFINITION

Usually taken to mean combined left and right heart failure. Most of the comments below also apply to pure right heart failure.

PHYSICAL SIGNS

The most important sign of right heart failure is elevation of the jugular venous pressure. Others such as hepatomegaly, peripheral oedema and cachexia occur in a variety of conditions.

CAUSES OF RIGHT HEART FAILURE

  – secondary to left heart failure
  – cor pulmonale (secondary to chronic lung disease)
  – rarer: cardiomyopathy, thyrotoxicosis, atrial septal defect, pericardial constriction, etc.

INVESTIGATIONS

Will be suggested by possible causes but must include:
Chest X-ray –note the heart size and look for signs of lung disease, pleural effusions, etc.
ECG
U+E – especially the potassium.

LFTs – especially albumin. Abnormal LFTs are common and improve with treatment.

Also consider FBC, thyroid function tests, echocardiography, and pulmonary function tests depending on the individual case.

MANAGEMENT

1. Rest, either in bed or in a chair.

2. Correct underlying abnormalities such as anaemia, hyperthyroidism, tachycardia and bradycardia. Stop cardio-depressant or fluid-retaining drugs. (beta blockers, NSAID etc)

3. Salt restriction – "no added salt diet".

4. Consider anticoagulation to prevent DVT or pulmonary embolism.

5. Aspiration of pleural effusions if large.

6. Diuretics: if failure is moderate or severe begin with frusemide 40–80 mg daily, increasing the dose as necessary, together with potassium replacements or a potassium retaining diuretic eg amiloride 5 mg daily. In mild failure begin with a thiazide diuretic eg. bendrofluazide K.

7. Digoxin – often beneficial even in sinus rhythm (see "Digoxin").

8. Vasodilators
   – isosorbide dinitrate 10 mg t.d.s. up to 40 mg q.d.s. especially if the patient also has angina.
   – prazosin 0.5 mg first dose in the evening, then 0.5 mg t.d.s. increasing as necessary.
   – hydralazine 50–75 mg q.d.s. or sometimes more up to a maximum of 800 mg/day. With the higher doses there is an increased risk of developing a lupus-like syndrome.

If the patient is on the above treatment and signs of failure persist, consider the following steps:

9. Change from potassium supplements to a potassium-sparing diuretic.

10. Increase the dose of diuretic.

11. Add metolazone 5 mg to the frusemide. This often produces a brisk diuresis but may cause marked hypokalaemia. Anticipate by increasing potassium supplements.

11. Dopamine or dobutamine infusion. For details see "Cardiogenic Shock".

The improvement is not long-lasting but it may be worth considering if the patient is not in end-stage cardiac failure.

Look for correctable lesions and refer for invasive investigation if necessary.

DURING TREATMENT MONITOR

1. Daily weight – more accurate than fluid balance.

2. Blood urea – often rises, especially in the elderly.

3. Electrolytes – low sodium when failure persists is an ominous sign. Watch potassium closely.

4. Chest X-ray – looking for reduction in heart size and to check the progress of pleural effusions.

Digoxin

Starting treatment:
Routine – 500 μg b.d. for 2 days.
    or – 250 μg b.d. for 7 days.
Rapid – 500 μg i.v. by infusion over 15 minutes.
    repeat after 1 hour, then 250 μg 4 hourly.
    or – oubain 250–500 μg i.v. slowly, then 100 μg hourly or oral digoxin.
    or – lanatoside 800–1200 μg i.v. then 200 μg 2–hourly to total dose of 1.5 mg in 24 hours.
Maintenance treatment:
    – in the range 125–500 μg/day.
    – reduced in renal impairment, old age, hypokalaemia.
    – serum digoxin concentration.
    – an inappropriately high blood concentration helps to confirm toxicity.
    – measure at 6–8 hours post dose.
    – normal therapeutic range 1–2 ng/ml (1.3–2.6 nmol/l).
    – check serum potassium at the same time.

DIGOXIN TOXICITY

    – more likely in elderly, renal failure, hypokalaemia, after diarrhoea and vomiting, after starting amiodarone.
    – produces nausea, anorexia, vomiting, xanthopsia, etc.

–ECG may show ventricular bigeminy, VT, multiform ventricular ectopics, atrial tachycardia with block, A-V block etc.

Treatment
1. Stop digoxin.

2. Increase potassium supplements (an infusion of 40 mmol in 1 hour can be given safely). Monitor serum potassium.

3. Give practolol 5–20 mg i.v. slowly for supraventricular tachycardias.

4. Use lignocaine for VT (see under "Arrhythmias").

5. Cardioversion can be used to treat VT when urgent restoration of normal rhythm is necessary. Start with low energy, such as 20 J, increasing if ineffective.

6. Give atropine 0.6 mg i.v. for A-V block or bradycardia.
    A temporary pacing wire may be needed.

7. Overdrive pacing of the atrium for SVT or ventricle for VT is often successful and can be repeated if the dysrhythmia recurs (see under "Temporary Pacing").

Antibiotic Prophylaxis Against Bacterial Endocarditis

Higher risk in patients with aortic valve disease, VSD, mitral regurgitation and prosthetic valves.
Lower risk in those with mitral stenosis, secundum ASD, "innocent" murmur.Many advocate no cover for normal delivery in pregnant women.

RECOMMENDED TREATMENT

1. Dental extraction, scaling etc.
       – 1 vial of Triplopen i.m. 30 mins before the procedure.
    or – amoxycillin 3 g orally 60 mins before procedure.
    or –in patients allergic to penicillin use erythromycin 500 mg
          orally 60 mins before and then 6 hourly for 24 hours after.

2. Genito-urinary procedures (sigmoidoscopy, cystoscopy, D+C) and abdominal surgery.
       – ampicillin 1 g plus gentamicin 80 mg i.m. 30 mins before

procedure or i.v. with the anaesthetic if given. Same dose of both drugs at 8 and 16 hours.

or – for patients allergic to penicillin give vancomycin 1 g i.v. (plus gentamicin 80 mg i.v.) by infusion over 30 mins about 30 mins before the procedure.

3. Patients with prosthetic valves
    – can be treated as above after 1 year.
    – earlier than that, consult the Bacteriologist.

4. Patients already on antibiotic treatment.
    – consult the Bacteriologist.

Management of Infective Endocarditis

INVESTIGATIONS

– always be suspicious in patients with murmurs or undiagnosed fever
– 3 blood cultures are usually sufficient (more if the patient has recently received antibiotics or following cardiac surgery)
– 4 hourly temperature chart
– FBC, ESR
– immunoglobulins, complement levels
– urine microscopy (for red cells)
– echocardiogram, looking for vegetations and for comparison later in the course of the illness.

If cultures are positive, the laboratory will measure antibiotic sensitivity and minimum inhibitory concentration (MIC).

If cultures are negative, repeat and also consider rare causes such as Q fever, psittacosis (diagnose on CFT) or fungi (check precipitins)

PRINCIPLES OF TREATMENT

Antibiotics and doses should be chosen in consultation with the Bacteriologist. High doses of bactericidal antibiotics are given intravenously and the course of treatment usually lasts six weeks, although in the later stages the drugs may be given orally. Great care must be taken to avoid infection at the site of the infusion. Subclavian lines are convenient, reduce the risk of thrombophlebitis and allow the patient more mobility. Probenecid is often advocated to increase blood levels of penicillin but makes drug rashes more likely and is probably best avoided.

Common organisms – Strep. viridans, Strep. faecalis, Staph. aureus (in acute endocarditis). Others are less common.

Commonly used antibiotics – benzylpenicillin, gentamicin, ampicillin, vancomycin (in patients allergic to penicillin), flucloxacillin.

During treatment monitor:

1. temperature 4 hourly

2. physical signs (murmurs, diastolic BP in aortic regurgitation,)

3. urine output

4. back titrations (in conjunction with the Bacteriologist)

5. renal function

6. Hb, WBC, ESR (anaemia and raised ESR may lag behind clinical improvement)

7. ECG (development of conduction defects is ominous)

8. chest X-ray (looking for any increase in heart size or sign of failure).

Persisting fever or recurrence of fever may be due to:

1. inadequate treatment

2. infection at the infusion site (remove cannula and send the tip for culture, including fungi)

3. drug fever (check for eosinophilia)

4. unrelated causes (urinary tract infection, DVT, pneumonia, etc.).

Systemic Embolism

CAUSES

 – mural thrombus in myocardial infarction, LV aneurysm
 – left atrial thrombus in mitral valve disease, AF, cardio-myopathy (note that emboli can occur with mitral stenosis in sinus rhythm)
 – aortic atheroma

– thrombus from prosthetic valve
– vegetations in infective endocarditis
– tumour in left atrial myxoma.

EFFECTS

 – cerebral: TIA, stroke, amaurosis fugax
 – mesenteric: pain, vomiting, rectal bleeding, peritonitis
 – renal: loin pain, haematuria
 – limb: pallor, pain, paraesthesiae, loss of pulse, weakness.

DIFFERENTIAL DIAGNOSIS

 – arterial thrombosis
 – arterial injury
 – DVT with peripheral vascular disease.

INVESTIGATIONS

 – blood cultures
 – ECG
 – cardiac enzymes
 – echocardiography looking for evidence of mitral valve disease, left ventricular disease, vegetations, myxoma
 – culture and histology of embolus removed at embolectomy.

MANAGEMENT

1. anticoagulate unless endocarditis or other contra-indication. May need to be delayed in stroke.

2. consider dextran 40 infusion.

3. angiography and streptokinase infusion may be indicated in renal emboli.

4. laparotomy may be necessary with mesenteric emboli.

5. in limb ischaemia, give analgesia and consider embolectomy.

Electrocardiography

1. Calibration. Normal paper speed is 25 mm/sec.
       5 large squares = 1 sec
       1 large square = 0.2 sec

1 small square = 0.04 sec
1 mV = 10 mm. Check this on each recording.

2. Standard 12-lead recording. The two commonest faults are transposed arm leads (giving inverted P waves in lead I) and chest leads all recorded on aVF.

    Chest leads are positioned as follows:

V1	4th intercostal space	right sternal edge
V2	4th intercostal space	left sternal edge
V3	over the 5th rib	between V2 and V4
V4	5th intercostal space	mid-clavicular line
V5	on horizontal line through V4	anterior axillary line
V6	on horizontal line through V4	mid-axillary line

3. Normal values

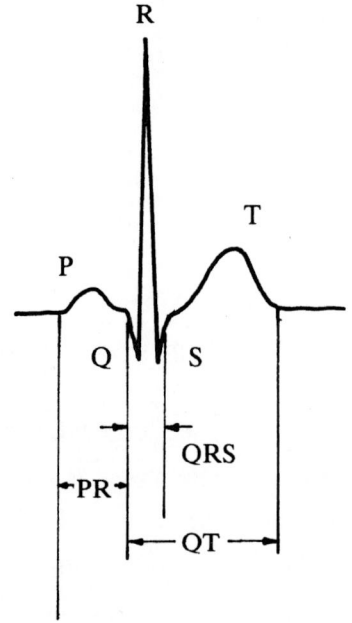

Figure 4

P wave <2.5 mm tall, <0.12 sec duration
PR interval 0.12–0.22 sec
QRS duration <0.10 sec
QT interval depends on heart rate
 <0.43 at 60/min
 <0.38 at 80/min
 <0.35 at 100/min

4. Rate. If regular count large squares between complexes
  2 squares = 150/min
  3 squares = 100/min
  4 squares = 75/min
  5 squares = 60/min, etc.
 If irregular, count the number of complexes in 30 large squares (6 seconds) and multiply by 10 for rate per min.

5. Axis. Normal range is −30° to +90° (or more in children).
 Left axis deviation is usually due to inferior infarction or left anterior hemiblock.
 Right axis deviation is usually due to anterolateral infarction or right ventricular hypertrophy or dominance.

6. P waves
  – look especially at leads II and V1.
  – bifid in left atrial enlargement
  –peaked in right atrial enlargement (congenital heart disease or chronic chest disease).

7. PR interval
  –short in Wolff-Parkinson-White syndrome and some nodal rhythms.
  –long in first degree block (ischaemia, digoxin, etc.).

8. Q waves – small 'q' is normal in leads I, aVL, and lateral chest leads with a horizontal heart and in II, III, and aVF with a vertical heart and is due to septal depolarisation. Deeper, wider Q or QS may be seen in aVR and V1 in normals.
  – abnormal if 0.04 sec or more in duration
    2 mm or deeper
    >25% of R wave in the same lead.
  –seen in infarction, pulmonary embolism, LBBB (in right precordial leads).

9. QRS
    - increased voltage in   (a) thin people
                              (b) ventricular hypertrophy
    - reduced voltage in   (a) obesity
                              (b) chronic chest disease
                              (c) myocardial infarction
                              (d) myxoedema
                              (e) pericardial effusion
    - increased duration in   (a) ventricular hypertrophy
                                  0.09–0.12 sec
                              (b) bundle branch block >0.12 sec.

10. Left ventricular hypertrophy. It is difficult to make a definite
    diagnosis on ECG unless the changes are very marked.
    Shows as (a) increased amplitude and duration
             (b) "strain" pattern in anterolateral ST segments and T
                 waves
             (c) left atrial hypertrophy.
    "Voltage criteria" -   QRS >30 mm in any lead
                           S in V1 + R in V5 >40 mm
                           S in V1 + R in V6 >37 mm

11. Right ventricular hypertrophy
    Shows as (a) right axis deviation

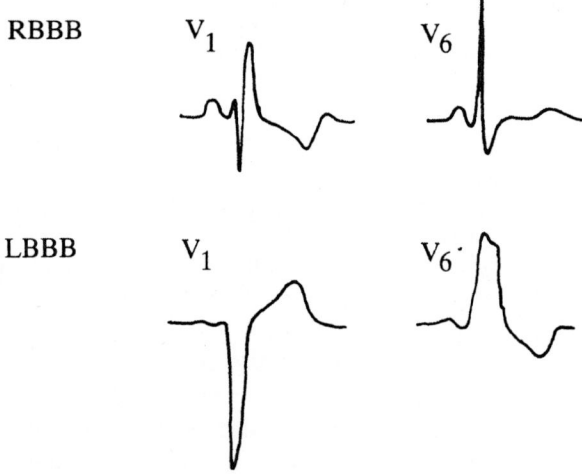

Figure 5

    (b) clockwise rotation

    (c) R > S in V1, R in V1 > 7 mm, S in V5 >7 mm

    Other causes of tall R wave in V1 are: incomplete RBBB, posterior infarction, W-P-W syndrome.

12. Left bundle branch block (see Fig. 5).

    Always pathological.

    It is usually impossible to diagnose ischaemia or infarction as well. Causes include ischaemia, hypertension, aortic valve disease, cardiomyopathy.

13. Right bundle branch block (see Fig. 5).

    Allows diagnosis of underlying infarction.

    Seen in normals, pulmonary embolism, ischaemia, ASD, conducting tissue disease.

    May be "incomplete" i.e. <0.12 sec.

14. ST segment.

    Depression in ischaemia, infarction, ventricular hypertrophy, bundle branch block, digoxin, hypokalaemia.

    Elevation in infarction, pericarditis, ventricular aneurysm. May be raised in normals or in LBBB in right chest leads.

15. T waves.

    May normally be inverted in III, aVR, aVL, V1, V2.

    Abnormalities are very non-specific and may be seen in many forms of heart disease and other diseases as well as being related to a variety of physiological activities (eg. hyperventilation, anxiety, change in body position, pre and post prandial.).

16. U waves.

    Best seen in V2–4.

    Inverted in anterolateral leads in ischaemia, and hypertensive heart disease.

    Prominent in V3–5 in hypokalaemia.

17. QT interval.

    Shortened by digoxin treatment and hypercalcaemia.

    Prolonged by ischaemia, infarction, hypocalcaemia, stroke, head injury, hypothermia, beta-blockers, amiodarone.

18. Electrolyte effects.

    Hypokalaemia – prominent U waves, flat or inverted T waves, ST depression, rarely first degree heart block.

    Hyperkalaemia – tall peaked T waves, smaller broader QRS complexes, small or absent P waves.

Monitoring Central Venous Pressure

INDICATIONS

1. Differential diagnosis and management of shock

2. Fluid replacement where the circulatory balance is precarious (heart disease, elderly, etc.)

3. Fluid balance in general anaesthesia and intensive care.

REFERENCE POINT

This must be defined and kept constant. It is usually either the sternal angle or the mid-thorax at the level of the sternal angle. Normal range depends on the point chosen. Recheck the zero if the patient's position is changed.

TECHNIQUE

1. Percutaneous puncture of the subclavian (either supra- or infraclavicular route), external or internal jugular or antecubital vein depending on your experience.

2. Insert catheter and advance until tip is in the lower SVC (but not in the right atrium). Check that blood can be aspirated easily.

3. Secure to the skin with a suture.

4. Connect to a saline or dextrose manometer.

5. Check that the column of fluid swings with respiration.

6. Zero the manometer with the chosen anatomical reference point.

7. Measure and record the CVP.

8. Arrange a chest X-ray to check the catheter position.

COMPLICATIONS

Mainly those associated with venous cannulation eg. thrombosis, septicaemia etc.

INTERPRETATION

1. high CVP
    - heart failure
    - overtransfusion
    - pulmonary embolism
    - superior vena cava obstruction
    - tamponade

2. low CVP
    - haemorrhage
    - fluid depletion   peripheral shutdown
    - dehydration

    - septicaemia
    - drug overdose   peripheral vasodilation
    - anaphylaxis

NOTE

The CVP is a poor guide to pulmonary wedge pressure in the presence of heart or lung disease or drug treatment.

A CVP line can also be used for drug infusion, i.v. feeding and blood sampling.

The trend of readings is much more use than an isolated recording.

Swan-Ganz Catheterisation

A Swan-Ganz catheter is a flow-directed ballon-tipped catheter which can be passed to the pulmonary artery without X-ray screening to measure pulmonary wedge pressure (indirect left atrial pressure and hence left ventricular filling pressure).

INDICATIONS

When monitoring of left ventricular end diastolic pressure (LVEDP) is needed, eg. in shock or pulmonary oedema when vasodilators are used.

Where repeated thermodilution measurements of cardiac output are needed.

To differentiate between VSD and acute mitral valve regurgitation following infarction (by multiple oxygen saturation measurements).

TECHNIQUE

1. Standard subclavian vein puncture as in "Temporary Pacing" leaving a plastic cannula in place.

2. Note the balloon capacity and prime the catheter with saline.

3. Inflate the balloon to check it is not punctured, and then deflate.

4. Advance the catheter 10–15 cm to right atrium (RA).

5. Inflate balloon. If X-ray screening is available it makes advancement to the pulmonary artery much easier but, if not, connect the catheter to a pressure transducer with an oscilloscope display and a continuous flush system of heparinised saline.

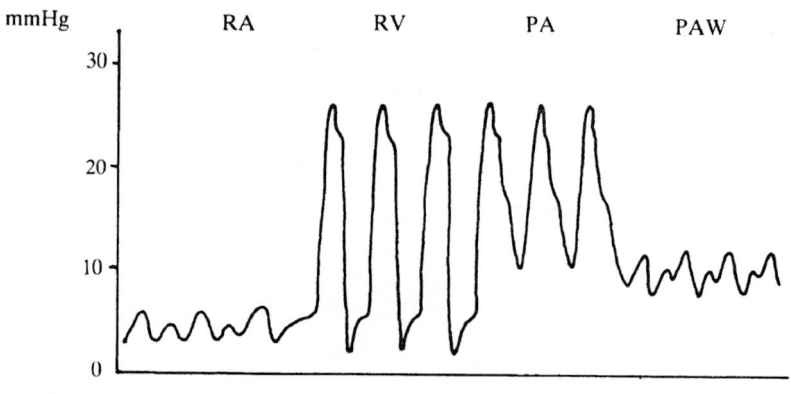

Figure 6

6. Note the RA pressure wave form (Fig. 6).

7. Slowly advance the catheter to right ventricle (RV) and identify by change in wave form (see Fig. 6).

8. Advancing the catheter farther should change the waveform to that of the pulmonary artery (PA) and then wedge pressure (see Fig. 6). If not pull back to RA and start again.

9. Once the catheter is in a position in the PA where inflation gives a wedge pressure and deflation a PA pressure, secure it to the skin with a stitch.

10. Apply sterile dressing.

11. Check catheter position with chest X-ray.

COMPLICATIONS

- those associated with subclavian vein cannulation
- balloon bursting: avoid overinflation
- catheter clotting: avoid by slow infusion
- pulmonary infarction: do not leave the ballon inflated in the PA
- failure to pass to the PA. Unusual, but may occur if the RA or RV are dilated, in which case X-ray screening is especially useful.

The catheter can probably be left in position for several days without problems but the latex does degenerate and the manufacturer will provide recommendations.

Temporary Pacing

INDICATIONS

- Stokes-Adams attacks before implantation of permanent pacemaker
- symptomatic bradycardia in acute infarction
- complete heart block or Mobitz II block in anterior infarction
- prophylactic in bifascicular block in acute infarction
- for overdrive pacing of SVT or VT.

PROCEDURE

1. Seldinger technique to cannulate the right subclavian vein (either supra- or infra-clavicularly). If not possible, try the left side. Alternatives are the medial antecubital or femoral veins but these are less convenient.

2. Introduce a 6F bipolar pacing electrode.

3. Using X-ray screening, position the tip of the electrode in the apex of the right ventricle.

4. Connect to the pacing box.

5. Pace on demand at 70/min (or faster if patient's own heart rate is over 70/min).

6. Slowly reduce the voltage to measure the threshold. Less than

1.0 V is acceptable, less than 0.5 V ideal. If higher than 1.0 V, reposition the electrode.

7. Check stability of electrode position by asking the patient to cough and breathe deeply.

8. Secure the electrode to the skin with a suture.

9. Apply a sterile dressing.

10. Leave the box set at 70 beats/min at 2–3 times the threshold (sometimes should be set slower or faster depending on the indication for pacing).

11. For overdrive pacing, the rate is set 10–20 beats per minute faster than the tachycardia rate to "capture" and is then slowly reduced until the rhythm returns to normal. Pace the right atrium for SVT and the right ventricle for VT. Ensure that the pacing box is capable of rapid pacing. Avoid sustained ventricular pacing at rates near or above 200/ min because of the risk of VF.

COMPLICATIONS

- those of subclavian vein puncture (bleeding, pneumothorax etc.).
- myocardial perforation is not uncommon. Normally does not cause serious problems. Recognise by pacing failure, friction rub, wire position on chest X-ray.
- pacing failure- ie. failure to capture or sense correctly. Check all connections. Review electrode position by X-ray screening. Reposition electrode if necessary.
- rising threshold. The threshold should be checked once or twice daily and will normally rise 2 or 3 fold over the first 7–10 days.

Conducting an Exercise Test

Despite the very small risk, all exercise tests should be supervised by a doctor. The commonest protocol is the Bruce test, which is performed on a treadmill with three min per stage.

Stage	Speed (mph)	Incline (%)
1	1.7	10
2	2.5	12
3	3.4	14
4	4.2	16
5	5.0	18
6	5.5	20
7	6.0	22

Before: explain the purpose and the procedure.
- record a 12 lead ECG lying and standing.
- measure BP lying and standing.
- ensure that the defibrillator is readily available.

During:
- monitor ECG, especially the rhythm and the ST segments
- measure BP at least once per stage.

Stop if:
- patient develops severe symptoms (pain, dyspnoea, fatigue)
- ventricular arrhythmias (other than unifocal ectopics)
- supraventricular tachycardia
- ST depression >4mm
- any ST elevation
- systolic BP falls
- the patient develops ataxia or dizziness.

Afterwards:
- monitor the ECG until it returns to the pre-testing record.
  note: the duration of exercise
        symptoms
        the reason for stopping
        the change in heart rate and blood pressure.

Contra-indications: heart failure, severe hypertension, severe aortic stenosis, acute myocardial infarction.

NOTE

– if VF óccurs, it is usually in the first few minutes after exercise.
– be prepared to admit the patient for observation if necessary (ie. prolonged pain or ECG changes, serious arrhythmias etc.).
– early post-myocardial infarction testing is becoming more popular as an indicator of prognosis. A much lower work load and a shorter protocol are used.

SUGGESTED READING

1.   L.H. Opie
     Drugs and the Heart. 1980
     The Lancet. London.

2.   L. Schamroth
     An Introduction to Electrocardiography 1976.
     Blackwell Scientific Publications.

2

THROMBO-EMBOLIC DISEASE

Deep Vein Thrombosis

CLINICAL FEATURES

Pain, swelling, increased warmth, discolouration, tenderness, oedema, prominence of superficial veins.

PREDISPOSING FACTORS

- immobility
- surgery or trauma
- neoplasia
- oral contraceptive pill
- polycythaemia
- age
- pregnancy

NOTE

A ruptured Baker's cyst can produce all the signs associated with a deep vein thrombosis in the calf, and should always be considered in a patient with any evidence of an arthropathy.

CONFIRMATION OF CLINICAL DIAGNOSIS

Unnecessary in many cases.
Venography is still the investigation of choice, although there is a small risk of causing a DVT.
Procedures such as the use of Sonicaid or doppler probes are frequently unhelpful as they tend to give positive results only in those cases where the diagnosis is obvious clinically, and may give false negative results if thrombi do not completely occlude the vein.

PREVENTION

- early mobilisation.
- subcutaneous heparin 5,000 units 12 hourly. In the case of surgery give the first dose 2 hours prior to theatre.
- anti-embolism stockings.
- pneumatic compression of the legs during surgery.

MANAGEMENT

General Measures
Elevate the leg, so the level of the foot is above the hips.
Support the leg with either bandaging or anti-embolism stockings.
Analgesics (not aspirin based).
Mobilise as soon as the acute symptoms have subsided.

Anticoagulation
Contraindications
- gastrointestinal haemorrhage
- severe hypertension
- cerebral haemorrhage
- bleeding disorders
- age. The use of anticoagulants, particularly long term oral anticoagulation in the over 65 age group is hazardous.
- early post-operative stage (24 hours) is a relative contra-indication depending on the type of operation.

Heparin
Give loading dose of 10,000 units i.v. then a continuous infusion in a dose of 20,000 units over 12 hours.
If facilities for continuous infusion are not available give 10,000 units by i.v. injection 6 hourly.
Monitor the effect by whole blood clotting time (normal 3–7 min) or APTT and aim for 2–3 times the baseline values. Dose required in range 30,000 to 50,000 units daily.

Warfarin
At least 48 hours is required before a significant effect is achieved from warfarin. If the decision to use warfarin is made, start early as

6–10 days are required before the patient's anticoagulation is stable.

– dosage: day 1 – 10 mg
day 2 – 6 mg
day 3 – 6 mg

reduce dose if the patient is known to be very sensitive to warfarin.

– check prothrombin time on day 4. Nomograms are available to predict maintenance dose depending on prothrombin time on day 4.

– aim for prothrombin time of 2.5–3 times normal

– continue for 6 weeks.

Pulmonary Embolism

MASSIVE PULMONARY EMBOLISM

History
– collapse, sudden dyspnoea, cardiac arrest.

Physical Signs
– hypotension, tachycardia, raised jugular venous pressure, right ventricular gallop, oliguria, cyanosis.

Investigations

ECG – may show: sinus tachycardia, low voltage, right ventricular strain, S1 Q3 T3, right bundle branch block.

Chest X-ray – may show: oligaemic lung fields, raised diaphragm, pulmonary infarction, small pleural effusion, or may be normal.

Blood Gases – reduced pO_2
– normal or low pCO_2

Lung Scan –perfusion defects with normal ventilation scan.

Pulmonary angiogram – shows obstruction of pulmonary arteries or filling defects.
– allows confirmation of diagnosis and assessment of severity.

Management

1. Oxygen in high concentration

2. Keep the patient flat (to increase RV filling pressure).

3. Avoid vasodilators (including opiates).

4. Heparin 15,000 units i.v. stat. then 30,000–60,000 units/24 hours controlled by whole blood clotting time or thrombin clotting time. Continue for 7 days.

5. If the patient deteriorates or if there is great haemodynamic embarrassment, consider the use of streptokinase:
    - give 600,000 units as a loading dose over 30 minutes
    - then 600,000 units 6 hourly
    - continue for 3 days then transfer to heparin
    - monitor pulmonary artery oxygen saturation and pressure during treatment.
    - the main complication is bleeding
    - the antidote for overdose is tranexamic acid 10mg/kg i.v. slowly
    - as streptokinase is antigenic, cover its use with hydrocortisone.

6. Embolectomy is available in some centres but is rarely indicated. It may be necessary in cases where anticoagulant or thrombolytic treatment is ruled out by recent surgery, active peptic ulceration, etc.
    Consider embolectomy if hypotension (systolic <90 mmHg), hypoxia (pO_2 <8 kPa), and oliguria (<20 ml/hour) persist after maximum medical treatment.

7. Maintain on warfarin for 6 weeks, or longer if previous history of DVT or PE.

MINOR PULMONARY EMBOLISM

This differs from a major pulmonary embolism in that pleurisy and haemoptysis are much more common and there is no significant haemodynamic upset.

Symptoms and Signs
Pleuritic pain, haemoptysis, dyspnoea, fever, pleural rub, pleural effusion.

Investigations
Chest X-ray – frequently normal but may show: linear or wedge shadows, raised diaphragm, pleural effusion.
ECG – usually normal
Lung scan – perfusion defects with normal ventilation.

Management
1. Analgesia

2. Oxygen if dyspnoeic

3. Anticoagulants (see DVT)

4. Reduction of risk factors (see DVT)

Reversal of Anticoagulation with Heparin

In many cases all that is required is to stop the heparin, since it has a short half-life.
Protamine sulphate is a specific antagonist (it has an anticoagulant effect of its own in excess).
Dose of protamine in mg = last dose of heparin divided by 200.
Give by slow intravenous injection to a maximum of 50 mg.

Reversal of Anticoagulation with Warfarin

If minor problems such as mild bruising occur, check PT and stop warfarin for 1–2 days then restart in lower dosage.
Bleeding; if minor and not responding to local measures such as compression, give vitamin K 15 mg i.v. slowly; if major bleeding occurs (eg haematemesis) give fresh frozen plasma in addition. Once vitamin K has been given it is impossible to anticoagulate with warfarin for up to 2 weeks.

Problems with Patients on Long-Term Warfarin

Many patients are on long term treatment with warfarin to prevent systemic emboli and stop thrombosis on artificial valves. Anticoagulation may need to be modified for:

1. Elective dental treatment; the dose of warfarin should be reduced to bring anticoagulation to the lower end of the therapeutic range prior to the procedure. For patients with abnormal or prosthetic valves antibiotic cover will be required in addition.

2. Emergency surgery; reversal of warfarin with i.v. vitamin K 2.5–20 mg slowly will be effective within a few hours. Patient with artificial valves will need to be re-anticoagulated as soon as possible post-operatively with heparin (warfarin will be ineffective for up to 2 weeks).

3. Elective surgery; stop the warfarin a few days beforehand and give i.v. or subcutaneous heparin. The exact level of anti-coagulation depends on the type of operation and the indication for warfarin.

3

RESPIRATORY MEDICINE

Respiratory Failure

DEFINITION

Respiratory failure is the inability to maintain normal blood gases. In specific terms if the pCO_2 >6.6 kPa (50 mmHg) or the pO_2 <8 kPa (60 mmHg) respiratory failure is present.

CLASSIFICATION

Type 1 Respiratory Failure – blood gases pO_2 ↓ pCO_2 ↓ or
NORMAL
Mechanisms – ventilation/perfusion imbalance
– venous admixture or anatomical shunt
Causes – left ventricular failure
– pneumonia
– asthma (may convert to type 2)
– pulmonary embolism
– fibrosing alveolitis
– adult respiratory distress syndrome
Treatment – increased oxygen concentration (35%+)
– IPP ventilation if reversible lesion
– treatment of underlying condition
Type 2 Respiratory Failure – blood gases pO_2 ↓ pCO_2 ↑
(a) Hypoventilation
Mechanisms – depression of respiratory centre
– primary alveolar hypoventilation
– mechanical factors (muscle weakness)
Causes – respiratory depressant drugs eg. opiates

        – neurological disease: Guillain-Barré syndrome
                              myaesthenia gravis
                              polymyositis
                              motor neurone disease

Treatment – maintenance of airway
               – removal of respiratory depressants
               – increased concentration of oxygen (frequently ineffective)
               – intermittent positive pressure ventilation

(b)   Ventilation/perfusion inequality in chronic bronchitis and emphysema

Treatment – removal of aggravating factors (infection and airways obstruction)
               – controlled increase in oxygen concentration (24–28%). Monitor CO_2 levels carefully.
               – respiratory stimulants, doxapram 1–4 mg/min i.v., only indicated if respiratory rate low.

Indications for Intermittent Positive Pressure Ventilation

Intermittent positive pressure ventilation may be required when other medical management has failed in:

1.   Hypoventilatory respiratory failure

2.   Mixed respiratory failure

3.   Where the patient is exhausted by the work of breathing eg. a prolonged severe asthma attack

4.   Left ventricular failure

5.   Post-operatively if the patient is unable to maintain adequate blood gases

6.   Adult respiratory distress syndrome

7.   Apnoea post-cardiopulmonary resuscitation

Administration of Oxygen

1.   High concentration – up to 60%
        – can safely be given in Type 1 respiratory failure
        – higher concentrations should not be used except for short periods

  – given via "Polymask" or "MC mask" with 6 l/min oxygen
  – both masks increase the inspired CO_2 slightly through rebreathing
  – humidification is probably not necessary
2. Low concentration – 24–35%
  – should be used in Type 2 respiratory failure
  – again, humidification is probably unnecessary
  – monitor response with arterial blood gases
  – give via
(a) Ventimask – the most accurate
    24% mask 4 l/min
    28% mask 4 l/min
    35% mask 8 l/min
(b) Edinburgh mask – more comfortable, less accurate
    1 l/min = 27%
    2 l/min = 30%
    3 l/min = 35%
(c) Nasal cannulae – best tolerated, least accurate
    1 l/min = 25–30%
    2 l/min = 30–35%

Adult Respiratory Distress Syndrome

This is a relatively new concept which describes a syndrome of severe respiratory distress occurring in a previously healthy person. A latent period of 18–24 hours frequently occurs between the triggering event and the onset of definite symptoms. There are clinical and pathological similarities to infant respiratory distress syndrome.

CAUSES
Aspiration, pneumonia, shock, severe trauma, drug overdose.
Exclude chronic pulmonary disease and left ventricular failure.
Must have clinical evidence of respiratory distress as shown by:
  – tachypnoea >20/min
  – laboured breathing
  – central cyanosis when breathing air
Chest X-ray – shows diffuse pulmonary infiltrates characteristically sparing the costophrenic angles
pO_2 – <6.6 kPa when concentration of inspired air >60%.

MANAGEMENT
  – IPP ventilation using a volume cycled ventilator

- positive end expiratory pressure of 8–15 cm of water (allows the use of lower concentration of inspired oxygen)
- antibiotics for specific infections
- methylprednisolone 30 mg/kg for 24–48 hours

Pneumothorax

Symptoms may range from nil to severe dyspnoea and pleuritic pain. The physical signs include:
- decreased movement of the chest wall
- increased resonance to percussion
- decreased breath sounds on the affected side.

Various clicks and pleural rubs may be heard throughout the chest and displacement of the trachea and apex beat may occur indicating mediastinal shift.

Causes
- spontaneous (commoner in tall thin young men)
- associated with chronic lung disease
- trauma
- rare conditions such as Marfan's syndrome
- iatrogenic (subclavian vein cannulation, pleural biopsy etc.).

Indications for the insertion of a chest drain in patients with a pneumothorax.
- tension pneumothorax
- dyspnoea
- co-existing lung disease (in view of limited respiratory reserve)
- bilateral pneumothorax
- large pneumothorax (>30% of lung collapsed)
- in patients who may require IPP ventilation.

Insertion of an Intercostal Drain

Equipment
- chest tube
- underwater sealed drain, tubing and clamps
- scalpel, stitch holder and strong suture material
- local anaesthetic.

1.   Assemble the underwater sealed drain checking all the connections.

2.   The normal site of insertion of a chest drain is in the 4th interspace mid-axillary line.

3. Infiltrate the chest wall with local anaesthetic down to the pleura.

4. Make an incision with the scalpel through the skin large enough for the tube to be inserted. Some blunt dissection of muscle layers may be required.

5. Insert two purse-string sutures around the incision, an inner and an outer.

6. Advance the chest tube under control. An obvious give will be felt when the pleura is punctured. Feed approximately 10 cm of tube, in the case of an Argyle catheter, towards the apex of the lung. Partially remove the stylet from the tube. Clamp the tube and completely remove the stylet. Pull the inner purse-string tight, and anchor around the tube. Connect to the underwater drain. Remove the clamps and the drain should bubble.

7. Arrange for a chest X-ray to check that the lung is expanding and the tube is satisfactorily positioned, directed towards the apex of the lung.

8. The patient should be asked to cough and breathe deeply to assist the expansion of the lung. The level of fluid in the tube in the underwater sealed drain should continue to swing with respiration.

9. If the tube stops swinging;
   – the lung may have expanded and blocked off the tube. Clamp the tube and arrange a chest X-ray. If the lung is fully expanded, repeat the X-ray 24 hours later and if the lung is still expanded remove the tube.
   – the tube may be blocked and require manipulation to clear it. Always clamp the tube before doing anything to the tube or the underwater sealed drain. Rotation of the tube or aspiration with a large syringe may clear the tube, otherwise it should be replaced.

10. If the lung fails to expand with the chest drain in place, gentle suction may be applied to the exit tube of the underwater sealed drain, just sufficient (10–25 cm of water) to stop the level of water swinging. Surgical intervention may be required if this fails to produce satisfactory expansion of the lung.

Pleural Effusions

Pleural effusions of more than 200 ml should be detected on a chest X-ray, more than 500 ml has to be present before the clinical signs (including dullness to percussion, reduced air entry and bronchial breathing at the upper border of the effusion) occur.

MANAGEMENT

Aspiration – sufficient pleural fluid for diagnostic purposes can be obtained without the need for a "formal" pleural aspiration, by the use of a 20 ml syringe and 21 gauge (green) needle. With the patient sitting forward, aspirate from the area of maximum dullness to percussion.

Fluid should be sent for
   – cytology
   – protein and glucose levels
   – Gram stain and culture including AFBs.
   – amylase (if pancreatitis or ruptured oesophagus are suspected)

Common Causes	Appearance	Protein Level	Other Features
Cardiac failure	clear	<30 g/l	
Tuberculosis	clear	>30 g/l	granulomas on biopsy culture occasionally positive, yield increases if large volume sent.
Post pneumonic	clear	>30 g/l	polymorphs
Malignancy	blood stained	>30 g/l	malignant cells on cytology. Recurs rapidly
Pulmonary embolism	blood stained	>30 g/l	
RA. SLE.	turbid	>30 g/l	lymphocytes, low glucose low complement in SLE. RW+ve in RA.

Formal Pleural Aspiration

1. Position the patient sitting forward with arms resting on a bed-table.

2.   Select the site for aspiration by clinical examination for the site of maximum dullness to percussion, and the chest X-ray appearances. The best sites are usually in a line below the angle of the scapula or in the posterior axillary line. To avoid damage to the intercostal vessels and nerves insert the needle immediately above the upper margin of the rib.

3.   Equipment
         – aspirating needles, large syringe and three way tap
         – receiver and dressing pack
         – local anaesthetic

4.   Infiltrate with local anaesthetic down to the level of the pleura. Connect the three way tap, syringe and aspirating needle.

5.   Advance the aspirating needle along the same track as the the needle used for the local anaesthetic, until a give is felt as the pleura is punctured. It should now be possible to aspirate fluid freely. All fluid that is aspirated should be measured.

6.   Stop aspiration if:
         – 1 litre of fluid has been aspirated, to aspirate further is to risk producing pulmonary oedema.
         – chest pain occurs.
         – haemoptysis occurs suggesting damage to the lung, which is rarely serious.
         – vasovagal collapse.

7.   When aspiration has been completed arrange for a chest X-ray.

Pleural Biopsy

This can easily be done at the time of pleural aspiration by substituting an Abram's biopsy needle for the aspiration needle.

1.   A small scalpel is required to make a skin incision large enough to take the biopsy needle.

2.   It is vital that the operator is completely familiar with the mechanism of opening and closing the needle prior to its use.

3.   Advance the needle in a closed position until it enters the pleural space, twist the trochar to expose the cutting gap of the needle.

4.   Engage the gap on the pleura in a downwards direction, the

direction of the gap being marked on the needle by a small raised bead. Close the gap by twisting the trochar and withdraw the needle.

5.   Repeat to obtain several biopsies.

6.   Arrange chest X-ray.

Asthma

Asthma can be defined as variable reversible airways obstruction and has several different symptom patterns:

Episodic asthma – frequently atopic.

Chronic asthma – usually non-atopic.

Nocturnal asthma – "early morning dipper" (after the pattern seen on respiratory function tests).

Corticosteriod non responsive – accounts for a number of the admissions to hospital with severe episodes.

Occupational asthma – described in connection with many industrial products, occurs on return to work eg. Monday mornings.

INVESTIGATIONS

Lung function tests – forced expiratory volume (FEV_1) before
                     – forced vital capacity (FVC)   and after
                     – peak flow rate   salbutamol

Chest X-ray – usually normal

Sputum – for culture, eosinophils and mycelia

FBC – eosinophilia

Immunoglobulins – IgE levels

Blood gases – in severe cases

Skin tests – if allergic bronchopulmonary aspergillosis suspected

MANAGEMENT

Patient mild to moderate symptomatically
     – Remove aggravating factors
                   ↓
     – Beta 2 sympathomimetic inhaler, salbutamol or terbutaline prn.

↓
– Beta 2 inhaler on regular basis up to 2 puffs 4 hourly
↓
– Add steroid inhaler, beclomethasone or betamethasone 2 puffs q.d.s.
AND/OR Sodium cromoglycate inhaler 1 spinhaler q.d.s.
↓
– Oral steroids.

Assessment of therapy – regular objective assessments in the form of peak flow rate or FEV_1 are important.

General treatment
– explanation of the condition to the patient
– stop smoking
– avoidance of obvious precipitating factors if feasible
– prompt treatment of chest infections
– desensitisation may have a small part to play in the treatment of patients who have specific allergies.

DRUG TREATMENT

Bronchodilators
The specific beta 2 sympathomimetic agents are the first line of drug treatment, salbutamol and terbutaline being commonly used, and most effectively given by inhalation. They can be used as required in those patients with occasional attacks or more regularly, up to 4 hourly, in those with more frequent attacks or persistent airways obstruction. When patients are first issued with an inhaler they should be supervised while using it, as many people, particularly elderly patients do not use them correctly, leading to failure of treatment. This may be due to problems co-ordinating breathing and manipulating the inhaler. Oral preparations, in the form of salbutamol 2–4 mg t.d.s. or terbutaline 5 mg t.d.s., are a poor second choice. They are less effective and have more side-effects. Slow release aminophylline preparations, such as aminophylline SR 225 mg b.d., are available for oral use, but tend to be limited in their use by gastric intolerance.

Prophylactic Treatment – Sodium Cromoglycate
In patients incompletely controlled on bronchodilators, sodium cromoglycate may be a useful addition. (Avoid using Intal Co which also contains isoprenaline). It is difficult to predict response to

treatment with sodium cromoglycate, so it is given a therapeutic trial for a period of 2–4 weeks and response is assessed at the end of that period. The initial dose is 1 spincap q.d.s., reducing to 1 b.d. if control is achieved. Less frequent use than this is ineffective, except in exercise induced asthma when it can be used immediately before exercise.

Steroid Inhalers

The use of beclomethasone or betamethasone inhalers 1–2 puffs q.d.s. allows small doses of steroids to be delivered locally to the bronchi without the side-effects associated with oral steroid treatment, but with an effect equivalent to approximately 10 mg of prednisolone. The only recognised side-effect is occasional oral thrush. When bronchodilator and steroid inhalers are used, the bronchodilator should be used first and 10–20 min allowed to elapse before the steroid is used in an attempt to ensure more effective inhalation of the steroid.

Oral Steroids

If possible, use short courses of treatment, eg. start with 35 mg of prednisolone daily, continue for 3–5 days then reduce by 5 mg daily until the course is completed. This produces fewer steroid side-effects than continuous oral steroids and is frequently very effective. In the older patient with late onset asthma, which may be confused with chronic bronchitis, steroids may be the only really effective treatment and a therapeutic trial of 30 mg daily of prednisolone for 14 days should always be considered.

For a small group of patients who require regular oral steroids attempts must be made to reduce the maintenance dose to a minimum, preferably less than 10 mg daily of prednisolone, although there is no safe dose.

Allergic Bronchopulmonary Aspergillosis

A small proportion of patients with asthma develop a hypersensitivity to aspergillus fumigatus, which may lead to the formation of bronchiectasis. The diagnosis is made by positive skin tests to aspergillus and precipitating antibodies to aspergillus in blood. Transient pulmonary shadowing and a blood eosinophilia may also occur. Treatment is in the form of corticosteroids and physiotherapy, and occasionally bronchoscopy may be required to remove mucus plugs.

Treatment of an Acute Asthmatic Attack

This is a condition with a significant mortality. Factors which are potentially capable of altering this situation include
- better education of the patient to recognise attacks
- early use of corticosteroids
- early admission to hospital.

ASSESSMENT OF SEVERITY

Features of a severe attack
- tachycardia >120/min
- pulsus paradoxus >10 mmHg
- recession of intercostal muscles
- severe breathlessness, too breathless to talk
- peak flow rate <100 l/min
- FEV_1 <20% predicted normal.

Features suggesting imminent need for IPP ventilation
- silent chest on ascultation
- cyanosis
- impaired level of consciousness
- pO_2 <6.5 kPa
- pCO_2 >6.5 kPa
- bradycardia
- hypotension (<90 mmHg)
- intolerable respiratory distress.

INVESTIGATIONS

Urgent
- blood gases
- chest X-ray to exclude pneumothorax and to look for evidence of infection
- peak flow rate.

Later
- FBC
- U+E
- ECG

TREATMENT OF SEVERE ASTHMATIC ATTACKS

1. Oxygen in high concentration 35–60%

2. Bronchodilators
   - Aminophylline in a loading dose of 250–500 mg (5 mg/kg), as a

slow i.v. injection. If given too rapidly cardiac arrhythmias and convulsions may be precipitated.

– Commence a maintenance infusion of aminophylline 0.7 mg/kg/hour which is approximately 500 mg of aminophylline in 1 litre of 5% dextrose over 12 hours.

– Nebulised salbutamol 5–10 mg in the form of a 0.5% solution may be administered by use of a Wright's or Hudson's nebuliser or by a patient triggered device such as a Bennett or Bird ventilator.

3.   Corticosteroids
     – ALWAYS indicated in severe attacks.
     – Hydrocortisone 4 mg/kg i.v. (approx 200–300 mg) followed by either repeated i.v. injections of 4 mg/kg 4 hourly or a constant infusion of 1 g over the next 12 hours.

4.   Antibiotics
     If from the history, clinical examination or chest X-ray, there is any evidence of infection one of the following antibiotics should be used;
          – amoxycillin 500 mg t.d.s.
     or – trimethoprim 200 mg b.d

5.   Fluid Intake
     – Correct dehydration which is frequently present.
     – Potassium supplementation may be necessary in view of the large doses of steroids being given.

6.   Mechanical Ventilation
     This should be undertaken in those patients fulfilling the necessary criteria (see assessment of severity), and should be undertaken as a controlled elective procedure rather than as a last minute emergency measure if at all possible.. Contact the anaesthetist early.

AFTERCARE

When the condition has been stable for a minimum of 24 hours, discontinue the aminophylline infusion and continue bronchodilators by inhalation. Replace the i.v. hydrocortisone with oral prednisolone:
     day 1 – 60 mg daily in divided doses
     day 2 – 50 mg

day 3 – 40 mg
day 4 – 30 mg

Continue to reduce the dosage of prednisolone by 5 mg daily, and stop if the condition allows.

Pneumonia

Primary – occurring in a previously healthy person
Secondary – occurring in association with:

1. pre-existing pulmonary disease
    – airways obstruction
    – carcinoma of the bronchus
    – fibrotic lung disease
    – bronchiectasis

2. viral infections,particularly influenza

3. aspiration

4. immunosuppression

CLINICAL FEATURES

Cough with or without sputum, dyspnoea, fever, pleuritic chest pain, crepitations, signs of consolidation.

INITIAL INVESTIGATIONS

    – chest X-ray PA and lateral
    – blood cultures
    – blood gases
    – sputum culture
    – sputum cytology

MANAGEMENT

    – oxygen in high concentrations (35% or greater) if the patient is hypoxic or distressed
    – correct dehydration
    – physiotherapy may help to clear tenacious sputum

Primary Pneumonias

	Organisms	*Therapy*
Primary Pneumonia	*Strep. pneumoniae* *H. influenzae*	amoxycillin 250 mg t.d.s. or trimethoprim 200 mg b.d.
Severe Cases of Primary Pneumonia		benzylpenicillin 2-4 mega units q.d.s. i.v. plus gentamicin 1.5 mg/kg i.m./i.v. t.d.s. (check levels)
Primary Atypical Pneumonia	mycoplasma legionella	minocycline 200 mg stat then 100 mg b.d. orally or erythromycin 500 mg q.d.s. orally

Secondary Pneumonia

Chronic Bronchopul- monary Disease	*Strep. pneumoniae* *H. influenzae*	amoxycillin 250 mg t.d.s. orally or trimethoprim 200 mg t.d.s.
In Suspected Staphylococcal Infection		add flucloxacillin 500 mg q.d.s. oral or i.v.
Post Influenza	*Staph. aureus* *Strep. pneumoniae*	benzylpenicillin 2-4 mega units q.d.s. i.v. plus flucloxacillin 500 mg q.d.s. oral or i.v.
Gram Negative Organisms		gentamicin 1.5 mg/kg i.v./i.m. t.d.s.
Aspiration Pneumonia	bacteroides species	benzylpenicillin 2-4 mega units q.d.s. i.v. plus metronidazole 400 mg t.d.s. orally and gentamicin 1.5 mg/kg i.m./i.v. t.d.s. (check levels)
Systemic Disease	varied	cefoxitin 1g t.d.s. i.v./i.m. plus gentamicin 1.5 mg/kg i.v./i.m. t.d.s.

Chronic Bronchitis and Emphysema

Chronic bronchitis is defined as cough productive of sputum on most days for at least 3 months of more than two consecutive years.

Chronic bronchitis is a spectrum with at each end a recognisable clinical entity, the "pink puffers" and the "blue bloaters".

Pink puffers – breathless, thin, not cyanosed with relatively normal blood gases.

Blue bloaters – obese, cyanosed, in right heart failure with clinical and blood gas evidence of CO_2 retention.

INVESTIGATIONS

Chest X-ray – may show flattened low diaphragms and a long thin heart, and if cor pulmonale develops there may be a change to an enlarged heart and dilated pulmonary arteries. Bullae.

Respiratory function tests – these are typically obstructive with reduced peak flow rates and reduced FEV_1/FVC ratio, an increased TLC and RV, and a reduced transfer factor.

Blood gases – used to quantify the degree and type of respiratory failure.

FBC – secondary polycythaemia is common and if severe may require treatment by venesection.

U+Es – renal impairment (due to poor perfusion) is common, and may be exacerbated by the use of diuretics, which may also induce electrolyte disturbances.

TREATMENT

1. Stop smoking.

2. Infection. Exacerbations require prompt treatment with anti-biotics such as amoxycillin 250 mg t.d.s. or trimethoprim 200 mg b.d. orally. It is often worthwhile providing patients with a supply of an antibiotic so that they can commence treatment as soon as they detect an exacerbation.

3. Bronchodilators. There is an element of reversibility in many patients. Salbutamol or another beta sympathomimetic inhaler may produce an improvement. A guide to the likely effec-tiveness can be gained from measuring peak flow rates before and 20 min after the use of the salbutamol. Some patients experience an improvement in exercise tolerance despite no

significant change in lung function tests. In addition the use of ipratropium bromide, an atropine-like agent, may produce a worthwhile response where the beta sympathomimetic inhaler alone has failed.

In an acute exacerbation intravenous aminophylline 4 mg/kg (250–400 mg) i.v. slowly may produce a degree of bronchodilation.

4. Steroids. Prednisolone 40 mg daily orally, or in an acute exacerbation,
    hydrocortisone 200 mg i.v. q.d.s. continued for 2 weeks, should be used to identify those patients with chronic asthma. If a significant improvement of lung function tests is not demonstrated at the end of that period the steroids should be discontinued.

5. Oxygen. This needs to be carefully controlled. A suitable method of controlling the concentration of inspired oxygen is to use a Ventimask, initially a 24% mask changing to 28% if 24% oxygen is tolerated without evidence of increasing CO_2 retention. Frequent blood gas estimations should be performed to monitor improvement in hypoxia and/or increased CO_2 retention. If the pCO_2 of a venous sample is measured at the same time as an arterial sample and the levels are compared, venous samples can be used to monitor changes in CO_2 levels, thereby saving frequent arterial sampling.

Bronchiectasis

Bronchiectasis is one end result of bronchial infection and should be considered in any patient with a cough productive of large quantities of purulent sputum, in any case of haemoptysis, with fibrocystic disease and immunodeficiency states.

INVESTIGATIONS

Chest X-ray – this may show cystic changes with fluid levels or tramline shadowing.
Respiratory function tests – an obstructive pattern is common.
Sputum – *H. influenzae* can frequently be grown on culture.
        Mycelia suggest bronchopulmonary aspergillosis.
Bronchography – this procedure is not frequently required but is the definitive investigation.

MANAGEMENT

– postural drainage twice daily at least.
– acute infective exacerbations require treatment with appropriate antibiotics depending on the results of culture and sensitivity. If these results are not available amoxycillin 250 mg t.d.s. or trimethoprim 200 mg b.d. orally will cover many of the likely organisms.

Lung Abscess

Lung abscess is a localised infection caused by pyogenic organisms leading to cavity formation.

COMMON CAUSES

– aspiration (frequently associated with alcohol excess)
– staphylococcal infection
– *Klebsiella pneumoniae*
– foreign bodies
– carcinoma of the bronchus

INVESTIGATIONS

– chest X-ray
– sputum culture and Gram stain
– sputum for AFB
– sputum cytology
– bronchoscopy

MANAGEMENT

Physiotherapy – postural drainage is most important and should be carried out at least twice daily.
Antibiotics – for aerobic organisms such as staphylococci or klebsiella cefoxitin 1 g t.d.s. i.v./i.m.
– for anaerobic infections benzylpenicillin 2 mega units q.d.s. i.v. or metronidazole 400 mg t.d.s. orally should be continued until there is radiological evidence of healing of the lesions.

INDICATIONS FOR SURGERY

– failed medical treatment
– empyema

- very large abscess
- uncontrollable haemoptysis

Haemoptysis

This is an important symptom which should always be sought and investigated if present. Despite this, no obvious cause may be found in up to 40% of cases.

CAUSES

- carcinoma of the bronchus
- pulmonary tuberculosis
- pulmonary infarction
- bronchiectasis and lung abscess
- pneumonia
- bronchial adenomas
- mitral valve disease
- thoracic trauma
- bronchitis
- Goodpasture's syndrome

INVESTIGATIONS

- chest X-ray PA and lateral
- sputum: culture, ZN stain for AFB and cytology
- bronchoscopy
- lung scan if pulmonary infarction suspected
- echocardiography if suspicion of mitral valve disease
- bronchography to determine the site and extent of bronchiectasis (prior to surgery)

Pulmonary Tuberculosis

Despite the fall in incidence of tuberculosis it remains an important condition as it is curable and the effects of missing the diagnosis are potentially lethal. A high index of suspicion must be maintained particularly in the elderly and in those immunosuppressed or debilitated by disease or treatment.

INVESTIGATIONS

- Chest X-ray

- sputum for AFBs
- sputum for TB culture (takes 6 weeks)
- Mantoux and/or Heaf tests. These are now less valuable because of the widespread use of BCG, unless strongly positive or previously documented as negative.
- investigations to exclude the presence of other underlying diseases such as diabetes

TREATMENT

Admission to hospital or continued stay in hospital is not required for treatment to be commenced unless the patient's general condition requires this or there are serious doubts about the patient's compliance. Infectivity is not a problem once treatment has commenced.

COMBINATION CHEMOTHERAPY

Drugs for the treatment of TB are always used in combination to reduce the problem of resistant organisms.
The Standard Regime
- isoniazid 300 mg daily (+ pyridoxine 10 mg daily)
- rifampicin: patients <55 kg 450 mg daily, patients >55 kg 600mg daily
- ethambutol 15 mg/kg daily.
Triple therapy is given for 2 months, then if the organism is sensitive to all three agents, stop the ethambutol and continue the isoniazid and rifampicin until the 9 month course is completed. In the case of resistant organisms or side-effects other drugs may need to be substituted.
- streptomycin 1 g daily i.m. (reduce the dose to 500 – 750 mg daily in patients over 40 years old or less than 50 kg)
- pyrazinamide 20–30 mg/kg daily orally.

PROBLEMS

1. Compliance – poor compliance is the commonest cause of treatment failure in patients with TB (the red urine in patients taking rifampicin may help to confirm compliance).

2. Some patients need a change in treatment because of the development of side-effects.

Drug	Contra-Indications	Cautions	Side-Effects
Isoniazid	drug-induced liver disease	impaired renal and liver function	sensitivity reactions neuropathies agranulocytosis
Rifampicin	jaundice pregnancy	hepatic impairment alcoholism	nausea hepatitis thrombocytopaenia induction of liver enzymes
Ethambutol	children optic neuritis elderly	renal impairment visual problems	optic neuritis colour blindness neuropathies
Streptomycin		renal impairment	hypersensitivity vestibular damage
Pyrazinamide	liver damage	renal impairment diabetes gout	hepatotoxicity nausea

Treatment of Non-Pulmonary Tuberculosis

The number of cases of non-pulmonary TB that now occur in developed countries is small. For this reason there are few large scale studies of the use of the short course treatment (9 months), using the more modern drugs, such as rifampicin. However there is no reason to believe that the shorter course of treatment will not prove effective.

SUGGESTED READING

1.   R.B. Cole
     Essentials of Respiratory Disease 2nd Ed. 1975
     Pitman Medical

2.   Sir John Crofton and A. Douglas
     Respiratory Disease 3rd Ed. 1981
     Blackwell Scientific Publications

4

NEUROLOGY

Meningitis

Meningitis usually presents as an acute febrile illness with headache, vomiting and photophobia. On examination the classical features are neck stiffness and a positive Kernig's sign. Patients who are immunosuppressed by disease or treatment may present with a less typical picture such as an acute confusional state, or drowsiness.

INVESTIGATION

Unless papilloedema or a progressive focal neurological lesion is present a lumbar puncture should be performed and the cerebrospinal fluid examined. Neck stiffness and drowsiness may occur in a patient who is coning due to the presence of a space occupying lesion. In this case the presence of focal signs such as a third nerve palsy would be expected. Therefore in the presence of such signs an emergency computerised axial tomography (CAT) scan should be arranged before the lumbar puncture is performed.
Collect 5–10 ml of CSF and arrange for urgent:
  – Gram stain
  – cell count
  – protein level
  – glucose
  – culture.
In some centres counter-current immunoelectrophoresis is available to provide rapid information about the type of infecting organism.
Also take blood for
  – glucose (for comparison with CSF levels)
  – blood cultures.
In all cases of meningitis a careful check should be made for the

presence of underlying infection such as chest or chronic ear infection, this being particularly true in the case of pneumococcal meningitis.

CEREBROSPINAL FLUID FINDINGS (N:Normal, P:Polymorphs, L:Lymphocytes)

Condition	Pressure	Appearance	Cells	Protein	Glucose	Remarks
Normal	60-150mm	clear colourless	0-5 lymph	0.1-0.4 g/l	2.4-5.6 mmol/l	glucose 60% of serum level
Meningismus	N	clear	N	N	N	sterile
Pyogenic meningitis	↑	turbid	500 + (P>>L)	↑	↓	organisms on smear or culture
Tuberculous meningitis	↑	clear to sl.cloudy	50-500 (P+L)	↑	↓	AFB on smear or culture
Viral meningitis	N or ↑	clear	100 + (L>P)	sl. ↑	N	viral studies
Cryptococcal meningitis	N or ↑	clear to sl.cloudy	100 + (L>P)	↑	N or ↓	yeasts on indian ink preparation

TREATMENT

1. as soon as the LP has been performed commence treatment with antibiotics
    benzylpenicillin 4 mega units i.v. 4 hourly and
    chloramphenicol 1 g i.v. 6 hourly
    changing to more specific treatment when the results of culture and sensitivity are available.

2. Intrathecal penicillin is not without risk and is unlikely to make a significant contribution to treatment and should not therefore be used.

3. If staphylococcal infection is suspected flucloxacillin 1 g i.v. q.d.s. is indicated in addition to the standard treatment.

4. In the case of meningitis associated with evidence of ear disease gentamicin 1.5 mg/kg i.v./i.m. t.d.s. should be added to the standard treatment. The levels should be checked and the dose adjusted as required.

5. Continue intravenous treatment for 4–5 days then change to an oral regime where possible and continue for 10–14 days in all.

6. Repeat lumbar puncture should be performed if the clinical progress is not satisfactory or if the diagnosis is uncertain.

7. Contacts of patients with meningococcal meningitis should be treated with minocycline or a sulphonamide.

Lumbar Puncture

INDICATIONS

Only if specific information is likely to be derived which would substantially contribute towards diagnosis, treatment or assessment of disease.
There are four main indications:–

1. Suspected infection by bacteria, viruses, fungi or spirochaetes.

2. Suspected sub-arachnoid haemorrhage.

3. Peripheral nerve diseases
   – Guillain-Barré
   – peripheral neuropathies.

4. Suspected multiple sclerosis.

CONTRA-INDICATIONS

1. Local sepsis.

2. Raised intracranial pressure as indicated by papilloedema, bradycardia.

3. Features suggestive of a posterior fossa tumour: drowsiness, vomiting, bradycardia, papilloedema.

4. Features of tentorial or tonsillar herniation: neck stiffness with dilated pupils, reduced conscious level and other features of a space-occupying lesion.

5. Suspected spinal cord compression.

6. If myelography or air encephalography are planned in the near future.

EQUIPMENT

Check that all the needles, three way taps and manometers fit each other. Needle sizes range from 18–21, the higher the number the shorter and smaller bore the needle. A number 19 is suitable for most adults.

TECHNIQUE

1. Explain the procedure to the patient.

2. Patients very rarely need to be sedated. This should be avoided if at all possible as the sedation may mask warning signs of deterioration after the LP.

3. Position the patient lying on his left side on the very edge of the bed. Flex the head and spine, get the patient to pull his knees up towards his chest. Place a pillow under the head and another between the knees. Ensure that the plane of the back is maintained in a vertical position.

4. Scrub up and wear sterile gloves.

5. Prepare the patient's skin with antiseptic and drape in sterile towels.

6. Locate the site of puncture by drawing two imaginary lines, one joining the tops of the iliac crests and the other running down the spinous processes. These intersect at the L3–4 interspace. A lumbar puncture can be performed at this space or one above or below.

7. Infiltrate the skin and interspinous ligaments with 1–2 ml of local anaesthetic. If larger volumes are used the local landmarks become difficult to feel.

8. Insert the needle exactly in the midline between the two spines, and advance it pointing very slightly towards the patient's head. A small "give" is felt as the needle passes through the ligamentum flavum. Withdraw the stilette and check for a flow of CSF. If absent try rotating the needle through 90 degrees; if no CSF is produced replace the stilette and advance the needle a few millimetres until fluid is obtained.

9. As soon as CSF is obtained attach the manometer, and measure the pressure in millimetres. The CSF should rise freely on inspiration and coughing. The normal CSF pressure is 60–150 mm.

Low pressure may be due to

(a) partial blockage of the needle

(b) blockage in the spinal canal or at the foramen magnum.

NEVER attempt to aspirate CSF using a syringe.

The Queckenstedt test shold NOT be performed to test for blockage.

High pressure may be due to

(a) a tense patient (up to 200 mm)

(b) raised intracranial pressure.

If the pressure is >300 mm

– remove the needle, the manometer will contain sufficient fluid for investigations.

– check the pupils, record size, symmetry and response.

– take the pulse and blood pressure and chart on a "head injury" chart.

– notify a neurosurgeon.

– if the pupils dilate, conscious level falls, or pulse slows, give 10% mannitol i.v. 500 ml over 20 min, and arrange urgent neurosurgery.

10. Disconnect the manometer and collect fluid for protein and glucose levels (also protein electrophoresis if MS suspected), bacteriology, serology (WR), and cytology if required.

   If the CSF is blood-stained, the appearance of uniform blood staining in 3 consecutive samples is strongly suggestive of a subarachnoid haemorrhage rather than a traumatic tap. The presence of xanthochromia in the supernatant also supports the diagnosis of subarachnoid haemorrhage.

11. Withdraw the needle and cover the wound with a small sterile dressing. After 3–4 hours if the patient is symptom-free he may get up.

12. Take blood for glucose level for comparison with CSF levels.

Cerebrovascular Disease

A SCHEME OF CLASSIFICATION

1. Vascular territory
   – carotid: hemiparesis, hemisensory, amaurosis fugax, language disturbance.

   – vertebrobasilar: vertigo, drop attacks, dysarthria, dysphagia, hemi or tetraparesis.

2. Stage of development
    – transient ischaemic attack, neurological symptoms and/or signs lasting for less than 24 hours.
    – completed stroke, focal neurological defects of vascular cause lasting more than 24 hours.
    – progressive or unstable stroke, changing pattern of neurological signs.

3. Vascular pathology
    – atherosclerosis
    – hypertensive vascular disease
    – aneurysm
    – embolism
    – arteritis.

4. Resulting lesion
    – infarction 80%
    – haemorrhage 10%
    – subarachnoid haemorrhage 10%
    – ischaemia.

5. Risk factors
    – hypertension
    – atherosclerosis
    – smoking
    – diabetes mellitus
    – polycythaemia
    – hyperlipidaemia
    – oral contraceptives.

INVESTIGATIONS

   – FBC, ESR, and platelets
   – chest and skull X-rays
   – WR or equivalent
   – U+E, blood glucose
   – ECG
   – urine testing.

Other investigations with particular indications
   – blood cultures if SBE is a possibility
   – fasting lipids profile in younger patients

- ANF if SLE is suspected
- echocardiogram if the lesion is thought to be embolic.

Definitive investigations
- lumbar puncture in suspected cases of subarachnoid haemorrhage in the absence of focal signs.
- computerised axial tomography
  indications
  - TIAs
  - to distinguish between haemorrhage and infarction prior to anticoagulation.
  - if the diagnosis is uncertain on clinical grounds.
- angiography
  indications - subarachnoid haemorrhage and carotid artery disease (only if surgery is contemplated ie. in younger patients without gross neurological deficit).

MANAGEMENT OF CEREBROVASCULAR DISEASE

Transient Ischaemic Attacks
The risk of a completed stroke following a transient ischaemic attack is up to 10% per annum.

1. remove or treat risk factors.

2. antiplatelet drugs – aspirin 300 mg b.d.

3. anticoagulants – only in a limited number of cases, particularly mitral valve disease and atrial fibrillation, or post myocardial infarction. CAT scan should be performed to confirm infarction rather than haemorrhage.

4. surgery, in patients with evidence of stenosing or ulcerating lesions in the carotid arteries.

Completed Stroke
In the vast majority of completed strokes no specific treatment required.
The exceptions to this are patients with cerebral haemorrhage (in particular those with cerebellar haemorrhage) who are admitted conscious and whose conscious level then deteriorates, in these urgent neurosurgical intervention to remove the haematoma is often

lifesaving. Other measures in the treatment of the patient with a completed stroke are directed at the prevention of further episodes by reduction or removal of risk factors and the prevention of complications.

Management
- maintain airway.
- adequate hydration, by nasogastric tube if unable to take fluids by mouth.
- good general nursing care is vital from the time of admission to prevent the development of pressure sores and hypostatic pneumonia which carry a significant mortality and morbidity.
- physiotherapy is important in the early stages to prevent the development of chest infections due to accumulation of secretions. Avoidance of development of contraction deformities should begin at an early stage by correct positioning of limbs and frequent passive movements, and at a later stage the physiotherapist has a vital role to play in the rehabilitation of the patient.
- avoid bladder catheterisation if at all possible as infection is inevitable.

Subarachnoid Haemorrhage

The diagnosis of subarachnoid haemorrhage is confirmed by lumbar puncture unless focal signs are present, when a CAT scan should be performed to exclude the presence of a large intracerebral haemorrhage before the lumbar puncture is carried out.
- treat risk factors particularly hypertension.
- keep the patient on bed rest until the symptoms have have improved, then gradually mobilise aiming for discharge after 2 weeks if no aneurysm is detected on angiography.

In patients who are under the age of 50 with an otherwise normal central nervous system and a normal blood pressure, carotid and vertebral angiography is indicated.

Coma

COMMON CAUSES OF COMA
- head injury

- cerebrovascular disease
    - stroke
    - haemorrhage
    - subarachnoid haemorrhage
- drug or alcohol excess
- epilepsy
- diabetic comas - hyperglycaemic or hypoglycaemic
- hypothermia
- space occupying lesions in the CNS
    - tumour
    - subdural haematoma
    - abscess
- CNS infections
    - meningitis
    - encephalitis
- systems failures
    - respiratory failure
    - renal failure
    - hepatic failure
- severe hypotension or hypertension
- if recently returned from abroad
    - malaria
    - other tropical diseases
- hysteria

MANAGEMENT

General Measures

1. Check and maintain airway with oropharyngeal airway, or if the gag reflex is absent, with an endotracheal tube. Turn the patient onto his side to reduce the risk of aspiration.

2. Respiration can be assessed quickly but crudely by the use of a Wright's spirometer, with the spirometer connected to an anaesthetic face mask. An inspiratory volume of > 4 l/min suggests adequate ventilation until more definitive evidence is available from blood gas results. Blood gases should be measured on admission
    - $pO_2 < 10$ kPa (75 mmHg)
    - $pCO_2 > 6.0$ kPa (45 mmHg)

    provide evidence of respiratory depression and indicate the likely necessity for intermittent positive pressure ventilation.

3. Look for and deal with other life-threatening problems such as severe hypotension.

History
Try to obtain a detailed history about the events leading up to the onset of coma from relatives, friends and any one else connected with the patient. A history of previous medical problems such as diabetes or epilepsy may obviously be important.

Examination
It is important to assess and record the degree of coma, and to record it in standard terms. One widely used method of recording the degree of coma is the Glasgow Coma Scale.
Eye Opening
- spontaneous
- to speech
- to pain
- nil

Best Motor Response
.- obeys commands
- localises painful stimuli
- flexion withdrawal to painful stimuli
- extension to painful stimuli
- nil

Best Verbal Response
- orientated
- confused conversation
- inappropriate words
- incomprehensible
- nil

EXAMINATION

Pattern of Breathing
Cheyne-Stokes respiration, a cyclical waxing and waning of respiration which is associated with:
- bilateral cerebral lesions
- brainstem lesions
- cardiac disease especially cardiac failure
- drugs eg. diamorphine.
Deep sighing respiration

- diabetic ketoacidosis
- mid brain lesions
- renal failure
- aspirin poisoning.

Irregular breathing
- medullary lesions
- pontine lesions.

Pupils

Unilaterally dilated fixed pupil
- implies tentorial herniation and is an indication for urgent neurosurgical intervention (check if eye drops administered)

Bilateral fixed dilated pupils
- poisoning with atropine or drugs with atropine-like effects eg.tricyclics, amphetamines, glutethimide
- advanced brainstem damage
- eye drops.

Small pupils
- opiates
- pontine haemorrhage
- pilocarpine eye-drops (in glaucoma).

Eye Movements

The so called "dolls eye" movement is an important response to elicit. The normal response to gently rolling the patient's head from side to side is a co-ordinated movement of the eyes away from the direction of movement. If this response is lost it suggests significant damage to the brainstem.

Fundi

Examination of the fundi may provide useful information in the diagnosis of coma.
- papilloedema suggests a space occupying lesion and is an indication for an urgent neurosurgical opinion.
- hypertensive changes
- diabetic retinopathy
- subhyaloid haemorrhage (in subarachnoid haemorrhage).

General Examination
- rectal temperature by low reading thermometer.
- neck stiffness,- suggests meningitis or subarachnoid haemorrhage.

- examine carefully for any evidence of head injury, including bleeding or CSF leak from ears or nose.
- skin lesions such as bullae in barbiturate poisoning, injection sites in drug addicts, and purpura in meningococcal meningitis.

Investigations
- Dextrostix for blood glucose (use foil wrapped ones as they tend to deteriorate and become inaccurate if exposed to air) or B.M. 20–800 sticks
- urine for glucose and protein
- U+E, blood glucose
- FBC
- skull and chest X-ray
- urine and blood samples for drug analysis, the exact availability of drug screening will vary from hospital to hospital but should always include barbiturates, aspirin and paracetamol
- further investigations will depend on the findings of examination eg. lumbar puncture in a patient with neck stiffness.
  Further management now depends on the underlying cause of the coma.

Collapse

Collapse is a frequent cause of presentation to the casualty unit and has many causes including:

1. vasovagal (simple faint) or variants of this:
    – micturition syncope
    – cough syncope.

2. CNS causes
    – TIAs
    – epilepsy
    – vertebrobasilar insufficiency.

3. cardiac causes
    – Stokes-Adams attacks
    – arrhythmias
    – myocardial infarction
    – aortic stenosis.

4. postural hypotension

  – autonomic neuropathy
  – anti-hypertensive treatment, particularly ganglion blockers
  – drugs with hypotensive side-effects eg.phenothiazines
  – haemorrhage.

5. hyperventilation and/or panic attacks.

6. pulmonary embolism.

Diagnosis of Brain Death

CONDITIONS FOR THE DIAGNOSIS OF BRAIN DEATH

All the following should co-exist:

1. The patient is deeply unconscious
    (a) There should be no suspicion that the patient's state is due to depressant drugs. An adequate interval of time (48 hours+) should be allowed for the persistence of drug effects to be excluded.
    (b) Primary hypothermia as a cause should have been excluded (body temperature should not be below 35°C before the diagnostic tests are performed)
    (c) Metabolic and endocrine causes of coma should have been excluded.

2. The patient is being maintained on a ventilator because spontaneous respiration had previously been inadequate or ceased altogether. Administration of relaxants, hypnotics and narcotic drugs must be excluded.

3. There should be no doubt that the patient's condition is due to irremediable structural brain damage. The diagnosis of the disorder must be fully established.

TESTS FOR CONFIRMING BRAIN DEATH

All the brainstem reflexes should be absent.

1. The pupils are fixed in diameter and do not respond to changes in light intensity.

2.   There is no corneal reflex.

3.   The vestibulo-ocular responses are absent. ie.eye movement does not occur during or after the slow injection of ice cold water into each external auditory meatus in turn, clear access to the tympanic membrane having been established by direct inspection.

4.   No motor responses within the cranial nerve distribution can be elicited by painful stimuli in any somatic area.

5.   There is no gag reflex or reflex response to bronchial stimulation by a suction catheter passed down the trachea.

6.   No respiratory movements occur when the patient is disconnected from the mechanical ventilation for long enough to ensure that the pCO_2 rises above the threshold for stimulating respiration, i.e. the pCO_2 must normally reach 6.7 kPa (50 mmHg). Hypoxia during the disconnection must be prevented as much as possible by delivering oxygen at 6 l/min into the trachea.

REPETITION OF TESTING

It is customary to repeat the tests to ensure that there has been no observer error.

STATUS OF DOCTORS CONCERNED

Normally the decision to withdraw artificial support is made by a consultant plus one other doctor.

Headache

TENSION HEADACHES
Tension headaches are very common and are related to muscle tension. They are described as a tight band around the head, which may be present intermittently, related to stress or may persist for months or years without relief. Many patients will respond to reassurance that there is nothing seriously wrong and to simple analgesics, while others prove resistant to all forms of treatment including anxiolytics and antidepressants.

MIGRAINE
A history of onset in the teens and a family history are common.

Prodromal symptoms are common, including flashing lights, fortification spectra, hemianopia, scotomata and paraesthesiae. The headache is typically unilateral and is associated with nausea, vomiting and photophobia in some cases.

Treatment of an Acute Attack
 – simple analgesics: aspirin 900 mg or paracetamol 1 g.
 – metoclopramide 10 mg oral or i.m. (if vomiting is a problem).
For severe attacks
 – ergotamine 1–2 mg stat orally and repeated once after 30 min if required.
 – ergotamine can also be given by aerosol inhalation in a dose of 360 μg repeated after 5 min if necessary.
 – it is dangerous to exceed the stated dosage, and the drug is contraindicated in patients with cardiovascular, hepatic or renal disease.

Prophylactic Treatment of Migraine
Patients experiencing severe recurrent attacks of migraine should be considered for prophylactic treatment. This should be explained to and discussed with the patient as "treatment failures" occur due to the patient not understanding the basic idea involved and taking the medication irregularly.
 – Pizotifen, 0.5 mg b.d. increasing gradually to a maximum of 1 mg t.d.s. if required, is frequently effective.
 – Clonidine, 25 μg b.d. increasing to 50 μg t.d.s. if required is an alternative.
 – In severe cases not responding to other treatment methysergide, 1 mg daily increasing to a maximum of 2 mg t.d.s., can be used.
 – Methysergide is contraindicated in patients with cardiovascular, renal, hepatic and pulmonary disease. Treatment should be withdrawn at the end of 6 months to reduce the risk of retroperitoneal fibrosis. A rising ESR may give early warning of this condition.

Incomplete Attacks
These attacks, in which headache predominates and prodromal symptoms are absent, frequently occur after periods of stress; if the stress is associated with work then they tend to occur at weekends.

Complicated Migraine

In this form of migraine transient, and very occasionally permanent, hemipareses and ophthalmoplegias occur. It is much more frequently associated with underlying structural lesions than the more common migraine variants, and because of this requires full neurological investigation including CAT scan. In contrast, simple migraine does not require any specialised investigation unless the onset is late in life or other features are abnormal. The use of ergot preparations in patients with complicated migraine is contraindicated, prophylactic treatment being the better course.

MIGRAINOUS NEURALGIA

This is a severe, strictly unilateral pain occurring around the eye. It is of relatively short duration, 15–120 min typically, and occurs most frequently at night in middle-aged to elderly men. A series of these episodes may occur over a period of a few weeks and then resolve, leading to the term "cluster headaches". Congestion of the conjunctiva, lacrimation and nasal stuffiness are commonly associated. The condition normally responds well to treatment with ergot preparations or methysergide in the same doses as used in migraine.

HEADACHE OF RAISED INTRACRANIAL PRESSURE

This is rare, often progressive and described as a dull aching sensation which is often poorly localised. It is worse in the mornings and is aggravated by coughing or straining. A headache which is severe or longstanding is unlikely to be due to raised intracranial pressure. Full neurological investigations including CAT scan are required in patients suspected of having this type of headache.

CRANIAL ARTERITIS

Cranial arteritis constitutes a medical emergency due to the risk of blindness. It occurs almost exclusively in older age groups, and normally presents as a severe persistent temporal headache. There may also be evidence of local scalp tenderness over the temporal arteries. Visual loss is the most sinister symptom as it is frequently permanent. A painful aching sensation together with stiffness and weakness of the proximal muscle groups, particularly in the morning, constitute polymyalgia rheumatica, a frequent association of temporal arteritis. The diagnosis is made primarily on clinical grounds. A markedly elevated ESR (>70 mm/hr) provides some supporting evidence but a relatively normal ESR does not exclude the diagnosis. Steroids in the form of prednisolone 60 mg daily should be commenced immediately and reduced gradually once the symptoms are controlled and the ESR starts to fall. Treatment with steroids should be continued for approximately 12 months at the lowest possible dose then gradually withdrawn. Temporal artery biopsy should be performed on all suspected cases of temporal arteritis, but treatment should not be delayed for it to take place. A normal biopsy does not exclude the diagnosis.

CERVICAL SPONDYLOSIS

In addition to the typical symptoms and signs in the upper limbs, occipital headache is a frequent symptom, typically described as radiating up from the neck as far as the vertex. The treatment is that of the cervical spondylosis: cervical collar, analgesia etc.

DRUG-INDUCED HEADACHE

A proportion of patients on treatment with indomethacin and possibly some of the other NSAIDs develop headaches which rapidly resolve when the drug is stopped. Any nitrates used in the treatment of angina may produce headaches due to vasodilatation.

SUBARACHNOID HAEMORRHAGE

MENINGITIS

Facial Pain

Pain may be referred from
- paranasal sinuses (infection or tumour)
- teeth (infection or malocclusion)
- temporo-mandibular joint
- eye (glaucoma)
- the heart to the jaw

TRIGEMINAL NEURALGIA

Characteristically brief severe episodes of pain in the second and third divisions of the trigeminal nerve, with associated trigger points. It may rarely present as a secondary condition in posterior fossa tumours and multiple sclerosis where it occurs in a younger age group than that normally found.

Treatment
- carbamazepine, 100 mg t.d.s. increasing to 400 mg t.d.s. in gradual steps if required.
- phenytoin, 300 mg daily can be substituted in patients unable to tolerate carbamazepine.
- intractable cases may require division by surgical or chemical ablation.

GLOSSOPHARYNGEAL NEURALGIA

The pain of glossopharyngeal neuralgia is similar to trigeminal neuralgia, but occurs in the back of the mouth or in the ear.

POST HERPETIC NEURALGIA

Some patients who suffer from herpes zoster go on to develop rather intractable pain and/or dysaesthesia particularly in the first division of the trigeminal nerve. Carbamazepine or phenytoin may prove effective. If not, a proportion of patients respond to stimulation of the skin either by vibration or by trans-cutaneous electrical stimulation.

ATYPICAL FACIAL PAIN

This is a diagnosis of exclusion, and may be associated with a depressive illness which should respond to treatment with an antidepressant.

Epilepsy

An epileptic fit is due to abnormal paroxysmal discharge of cerebral neurones. A single epileptic fit does not constitute epilepsy, which is a continuing tendency to fits. In making a diagnosis of epilepsy the history is the most important feature, and as much information as possible should be obtained from relatives, friends or any other witnesses to the event.

GENERALISED SEIZURES

Petit Mal
Short absences, with no associated features, which only appear in children. They have a typical 3 per sec. spike and wave activity on EEG.

Grand Mal (Tonic Clonic Seizures)

An aura occurs in approximately half the cases. This is followed by the tonic phase lasting up to 30 sec, which then converts to a clonic phase. Injuries may occur due to the fall or in the clonic phase and unless the patient is in an obviously dangerous situation, he should be left alone. Attempting to insert things into the patient's mouth only leads to damage to teeth and gums, and bitten fingers. Patients are frequently incontinent of urine and less frequently of faeces. They typically remain unconscious for periods of up to 30 min and may then sleep for several hours. Plantar responses are extensor during the attack and remain so for some time afterwards.

Temporal Lobe Epilepsy

May present in a variety of forms. The patient may appear dazed and unresponsive, chewing or lip-smacking or more complex motor activity can occur. A generalised convulsion may be the conclusion of the attack in some cases. A sensation of familiarity with surroundings, dejà vu , or unfamiliarity, jamais vu, may be a feature.

FOCAL SEIZURES

Jacksonian Epilepsy

Occurs when there is a localised lesion in the motor cortex. It starts with a localised convulsion often affecting the hand, which then spreads or "marches" and may become generalised. A transient weakness may occur in the involved limbs after the episode, known as a "Todd's" paralysis.

INVESTIGATIONS

A single fit does not normally require investigation unless there are obvious focal features present.
- FBC and ESR
- blood glucose
- WR or equivalent
- chest and skull X-rays
- EEG

If there is any evidence of focal features, either clinically or on EEG, a CAT scan should be performed.

MANAGEMENT

1. Patient education – it is important to explain the diagnosis to the

patient as there are many misconceptions and fears about epilepsy in the population. Driving and epilepsy – a driving licence may be issued if the patient has been free from fits for 3 years. Nocturnal fits alone are not counted for these purposes.

2. Drug Treatment – general principles
    (a) commence only when the patient has had more than one fit
    (b) use a single anticonvulsant and increase the dose to achieve therapeutic levels before changing drugs.
    (c) change only one medication at a time. Add it to the existing regime and then tail off the failed drug.
    (d) monitor drug levels
    (e) when the patient has been completely free of fits for 3 years, consider tailing off treatment but discuss this with him first as some prefer to stay on treatment rather than face the slightly higher risk of having another fit.

3. Drug Treatment – specifics
    Grand mal epilepsy:
            1. phenytoin
            2. carbamazepine
            3. sodium valproate
    Temporal lobe epilepsy:
            1. carbamazepine
            2. phenytoin
    Petit mal epilepsy:
            1. sodium valproate
            2. ethosuximide

    Phenytoin: 300 mg daily increasing in steps of 25–50 mg to a maximum of 600 mg daily depending on blood levels and clinical response. Therapeutic range 10–20 μg/ml

    Carbamazepine: 100 mg b.d. increasing to 400 mg t.d.s. depending on levels and clinical response. Therapeutic range 5–12 μg/ml

    Sodium valproate: 200 mg t.d.s. to 800 mg t.d.s. Therapeutic range 50–100 μg/ml

    Ethosuximide: 500 mg daily to 2.0 g daily. Therapeutic range 50–100 μg/ml.

Status Epilepticus

DEFINITION

Recurring epileptic fits without recovery of consciousness between fits or a single continuous fit lasting for longer than one hour. This is a medical emergency with a significant mortality and should be managed where facilities are at hand for intermittent positive pressure ventilation.

TREATMENT

1. Diazepam 10 mg i.v. over 5 min.
    Repeat until convulsions are controlled or until a dose of 60 mg has been given or respiratory problems are encountered.

2. Once controlled switch to a diazepam infusion (40 mg added to 500ml of N saline), at 1–2 mg/hour increasing to 8 mg/hour if necessary (max dose 3 mg/kg/24 hours).

3. If the diazepam fails to control the fits:
    Chlormethiazole 40–100 ml of a 0.8% solution should be given as an i.v. infusion over 3–5 min to control the fits then the rate of infusion reduced to a maintenance dose, usually 10–40 ml/hour.

4. If control is still not achieved: Use thiopentone 25–100 mg i.v. slowly until the convulsions cease. Then switch to an i.v. infusion of 1 g of thiopentone in 500 ml of 5% dextrose at a rate of 0.5 to 1 ml/min. The patient will almost certainly require IPP ventilation if barbiturates are being used.

5. Once the patient's condition is stable:
    (a) if previously untreated give phenytoin 1g stat then 400 mg daily via nasogastric tube if necessary.
    (b) if already on treatment, measure drug levels then resume treatment if suitable in higher dosage.

6. A significant number of patients who develop status epilepticus have an underlying structural lesion and all should undergo full neurological investigation including CAT scan.

7. In the group of patients with no history of previous epilepsy approximately 20% will have taken a drug overdose and 10% will have an underlying metabolic problem eg. hypoglycaemia, hypernatraemia, hypocalcaemia, hypomagnesaemia, hyperosmolarity, vitamin B_6 deficiency, myxoedema, renal and liver failure.

Parkinson's Syndrome

CLINICAL FEATURES

- tremor, present at rest and decreased by movement.
- rigidity of cogwheel type.
- immobile facies.
- bradykinesia.
- stooping shuffling gait with lack of associated arm movements.
- impaired postural and righting reflexes.

MANAGEMENT

General Measures
- withdraw any drugs which may have precipitated the syndrome. (eg phenothiazines)
- physiotherapy and occupational therapy help to maximise the functional improvement achieved with the aid of drugs.

Drug Treatment
For patients with a significant disability, levodopa in conjunction with a peripheral dopa decarboxylase inhibitor, is the drug of choice. In patients with milder disability, particularly tremor or rigidity rather than bradykinesia, anticholinergic drugs may be useful. A beta-blocker may be useful in reducing tremor if this is a particular problem. Drug-induced Parkinsonism should be treated with anticholinergic drugs.

1. L.Dopa with the dopa decarboxylase inhibitor carbidopa (Sinemet)
    - start in low dose eg. Sinemet 110 1/2 a tablet daily.
    - increase over a week to Sinemet 110 1 tablet b.d.
    - this may be all that is required to produce a significant effect; if so continue at this dose.
    - increase the dose by one tablet per week of Sinemet 110, until a dose of two tabs t.d.s. is reached, then switch to Sinemet 275, one tab t.d.s.. The maximum dose is six Sinemet 275 daily, although side-effects may have prevented an increase in dosage before this level is reached.
    - side-effects include upper GIT symptoms, agitation, insomnia, vivid dreams, involuntary movements, and postural hypotension.

2. Anticholinergics
   – benzhexol 2–5 mg t.d.s. or
   – orphenadrine 50–100 mg q.d.s.
   side-effects are dry mouth, blurred vision, urinary retention and confusion.

3. Amantadine
   – useful in some patients unable to tolerate L.dopa.
   – 100 mg daily increasing to 200 mg daily after 1 week.
   – response occurs within 2 weeks.

4. Bromocryptine
   – useful in some patients unable to tolerate L.dopa.
   – 1.25 mg at night with food increasing gradually to 40 mg daily if necessary.

Myasthenia Gravis

Diagnosis is made from a characteristic history of fatiguability and weakness particularly affecting the extra-ocular muscles and bulbar muscles. It can be confirmed by a Tensilon (edrophonium) test.

TENSILON TEST

Before starting the test select an involved area, eg. ptosis, and use that as a baseline from which to judge the effect of the drug.
Give 1 mg of edrophonium followed by the rest of the 10 mg ampoule if no side-effects have occurred.
A positive response is indicated by an obvious improvement within 1 min lasting 3–5 min.
Unpleasant side-effects can be rapidly abolished by atropine 0.6 mg i.v. stat.

INVESTIGATIONS

- chest X-ray PA and lateral
- tomography of anterior mediastinum or
- CAT scan of mediastinum

looking for evidence of a thymoma

TREATMENT

– neostigmine 15 mg 4 hourly increasing to 30 mg 2 hourly if required.

- at the higher doses atropine 0.6 mg b.d. may be required to reduce some of the muscarinic effects.
- pyridostigmine has a weaker but more prolonged action of up to 6 hours, dosage 60 mg 6 hourly to 120 mg 3 hourly.
- steroids may be necessary in some resistant cases, but are not without risks. Prednisolone 60 mg on alternate days is a good compromise between effect and side-effect.

MYASTHENIC CRISIS

A severe exacerbation of myasthenic weakness which may be precipitated by the stress of infection or trauma.

Treatment
- Ventilation. Monitor frequently with a Wright's spirometer, if minute volume falls below 4 l/min check blood gases immediately and prepare for possible use of ventilation. If pO_2 <10 kPa (75 mmHg) or pCO_2 >6.5 kPa (50 mmHg), ventilation is required.
- Anticholinesterase therapy. Neostigmine 1–2.5 mg s.c. or i.m., the effect lasting for 4–6 hours.
- If the patient fails to respond immunosuppressants or, in some centres plasmaphoresis, should be considered.

CHOLINERGIC CRISIS

A cholinergic crisis is a rare problem and is due to over-treatment with anticholinesterase drugs. The symptoms include colic, sweating and fasciculation, proceeding to confusion and coma if severe.

Treatment
- monitor and maintain respiration.
- stop anticholinesterase drugs.
- atropine 0.6 mg s.c. blocks the muscarinic effects of the excess anticholinesterases.

NOTE

If in doubt as to the cause of problems in a patient with myasthenia, either myasthenic or cholinergic crisis, use the Tensilon test to distinguish between them. In a myasthenic crisis the patient given Tensilon will improve, in the case of a cholinergic crisis there will be no change or a transient (2–3 min) deterioration.

Guillain-Barré Syndrome (Acute Infective Polyneuritis)

CLINICAL FEATURES

Acute onset of paraesthesiae and /or pain in the extremities, followed by increasing muscle weakness, proximal as well as distal, and in severe cases involving the respiratory and bulbar muscles. The maximum disability is reached within 3 weeks, often much sooner. Cranial nerve lesions including facial nerve palsies (unilateral or bilateral) and III, IV and VI nerve lesions are often present.

Respiratory and bulbar involvement leads to the mortality which is associated with this condition.

INVESTIGATIONS

- viral studies.
- ECG (arrhythmias associated with autonomic involvement may be present).
- lumbar puncture (protein markedly increased, no increase in cells. For details see CSF findings).
- nerve conduction studies, abnormal with marked slowing of motor conduction associated with segmental demyelination.
- a proportion of cases are associated with malignancy, so it is wise to investigate this possibility in older patients and atypical cases.

MANAGEMENT

1. In many cases the course of the condition is relatively benign, and only requires general nursing care of a patient with muscle weakness, with mobility of the joints being maintained and remaining muscle power being exercised regularly. A complete recovery can be expected over the course of a few months .

2. In patients having difficulty in coughing effectively due to weakness, regular chest physiotherapy is required to help patients clear bronchial secretions, which would otherwise predispose to infection.

3. If problems with secretions continue despite chest physiotherapy a tracheostomy is indicated.

4. If major bronchi become blocked bronchoscopy is an effective method of clearing them.

5.   The great danger of this condition is hypoventilatory respiratory failure due to involvement of the respiratory muscles. This may be difficult to detect on purely clinical grounds as the patient frequently does not appear distressed. Respiration should be monitored with peak flow rates and minute volumes by a Wright's spirometer.

6.   If the peak flow rate falls below 100 l/min or the minute volume below 4 l/min measure blood gases and consider a tracheostomy. It is far better to do a tracheostomy as an elective procedure than to deal with a patient who needs ventilating as an emergency.

7.   Blood gases of pO_2 <10 kPa, pCO_2 >6.5 kPa are indications for ventilation particularly if the trend of the blood gases is worsening.

8.   If bulbar problems occur during feeding, the patient should be fed through a nasogastric tube.

9.   ACTH 60 units daily may be helpful in the early stages in some patients. Gradually reduce the frequency and dosage aiming to discontinue after 4–5 weeks, or earlier if no obvious response is achieved.

10. Severely affected patients who are immobile for long periods of time are at risk of developing deep vein thromboses and subsequent pulmonary emboli. To reduce this risk heparin 5000 units b.d. is indicated as a prophylactic measure but must be started early to be effective.

Acute Confusional State

An acute confusional state is the impairment of the higher centres of the brain leading to reduced attention, increased distractability, restlessness, irritability and disorientation in time and space.

CAUSES

1.   infection
        – septicaemia
        – chest infection
        – urinary tract infection
     This occurs particularly in the older patient in whom other signs of infection may be minimal.

2. drugs
    – some drugs, in what are normally therapeutic doses, may cause confusion, particularly in the elderly eg. benzodiazepines.
    – when drugs such as barbiturates or amphetamines are misused, or psychotropic drugs such as LSD are taken, patients may be seen in the casualty department in an acute confusional state during or after a "bad trip".

3. alcohol excess or withdrawal states.
4. diabetic problems
    – hypoglycaemia may present as a confusional state particularly in the elderly patient on long acting agents.

5. hypo or hyperthyroidism; in the elderly the clinical signs of hyperthyroidism may be minimal.

6. electrolyte disturbances eg. hypo or hypernatraemia.

7. disturbances of water balance eg. inappropriate ADH secretion, dehydration.

8. CNS disorders
    – infection (meningitis, encephalitis)
    – small stroke
    – subdural haematoma
    – post-ictal states.

9. psychiatric problems
    – acute schizophrenia (restlessness, paranoid delusions, auditory hallucinations)
    – acute mania.

10. vitamin deficiencies
    – B_{12}
    – Wernicke's encephalopathy.

INVESTIGATIONS

    – FBC, ESR.
    – U+E, LFTs, blood glucose.
    – GGT (good indicator of alcohol induced liver damage).
    – blood cultures.
    – B_{12}, WR.
    – T_4, FTI.

– routine urine testing plus MSU.
– chest and skull X-ray.

MANAGEMENT

The major objective is to identify and correct the underlying cause. Sedation of confused patients should be avoided if possible but, if necessary for the safety of the patient and/or staff, chlorpromazine should be given (initially in small doses eg. 25–50 mg orally or i.m. increasing to 150 mg if necessary).
Haloperidol 1–5 mg orally or in an emergency 5–10 mg i.v. is an alternative.

Dementia

DEFINITION

A diffuse deterioration in higher mental function, particularly intellect, behaviour and personality.

TREATABLE CAUSES

1. Metabolic
        – hypothyroidism
        – hypopituitarism
        – hypercalcaemia
        – hepatic encephalopathy
        – uraemia

2. Deficiency states
        – vitamin B_{12}
        – vitamin B complex B_1, B_6.

3. Drugs
        – barbiturates
        – amphetamines
        – bromides

4. Alcohol

5. Infections
        – neurosyphilis
        – encephalitis
        – chronic meningitis

6. Trauma
    – subdural haematoma

7. Neoplasms
    – particularly frontal lobe

8. Obstructive or communicating hydrocephalus

9. Multiple emboli

10. Systemic lupus erythematosus.

NON-TREATABLE CAUSES

1. Alzheimer's disease

2. Pick's disease

3. Huntington's chorea

4. Jacob-Creutzfeldt disease

5. Arteriosclerosis

6. Multiple sclerosis

7. Parkinson's disease

INVESTIGATIONS

Routine
- FBC, ESR (may be macrocytosis in B_{12} deficiency).
- U+E and LFTs.
- VDRL.
- B_{12}.
- T_4, TBG, TSH.
- Chest and skull X-ray.
- Computerised axial tomography (has improved the accuracy of diagnosis and must now be included in the "routine" list of investigations of dementia).

Selective
- CSF if chronic meningitis or neurosyphilis suspected.
- EEG may give evidence of diffuse or focal nature of lesions.
- carotid angiography looking for evidence of carotid or cerebrovascular disease.

SUGGESTED FURTHER READING

1.   J. Patten (1977).
      Neurological Differential Diagnosis
      Harold Starke Ltd

 2.   Sir Roger Bannister (1978).
      Brain's Clinical Neurology 5th Ed.
      Oxford Medical Publications

5

LIVER DISEASE

Liver Failure

Liver failure may be acute (eg. post viral hepatitis) or may occur against the background of established disease (eg. cirrhosis).

INVESTIGATIONS

–FBC, platelets, prothrombin time
–U+E, LFTs, blood glucose
–Blood cultures and ascitic fluid for culture
–Hepatitis B antigens.

MANAGEMENT OF LIVER FAILURE

1. Treat or remove precipitating factors including: haemorrhage, infection, alcohol, drugs and electrolyte disturbances.

2. Commence a protein-free, high carbohydrate diet, re-introducing protein as the patient's condition improves. Hypoglycaemia is not uncommon in patients with liver failure and requires correction.

3. Give lactulose initially 30–50 ml 8 hourly until diarrhoea develops and then reduce dosage to produce 2–3 loose motions daily.

4. Neomycin 1 g q.d.s. orally.

5. Correct fluid balance. If oedema is present reduce fluid intake to 1 l daily or further if no response is produced. A diuretic is occasionally required eg. spironolactone commencing with a dose of 25 mg b.d. and increasing with care.

6. Electrolytes. Hypokalaemia is often present and needs correcting with potassium supplements. (Avoid using spironolactone and potassium supplements concurrently as hyperkalaemia can occur).
    Hyponatraemia is a reflection of fluid overload not sodium depletion and should correct with diuretics. Do not give N.saline.

7. Attempt to correct the haemorrhagic tendency with vitamin K and fresh frozen plasma, either when haemorrhage is a problem or to allow diagnostic procedures such as liver biopsy to be undertaken.

8. Cimetidine 200 mg t.d.s. and 400 mg nocte helps to prevent gastric erosions.

Bleeding Varices

This should be suspected where bleeding from the upper gastrointestinal tract occurs in patients with obvious liver disease, although even then the bleeding is more frequently from gastric erosions. Endoscopy is required to confirm the diagnosis.

MANAGEMENT

In the initial stages the management is as for any upper GIT bleed with the addition of the following:

1. Correction of clotting defects
    – fresh frozen plasma 1 unit as soon as possible then repeat after every 2–3 units of blood given.
    – vitamin K 15 mg i.v.
    – calcium gluconate, 10 ml of 10% solution to correct the effects of citrate after 4 units of blood have been given.

2. Control of bleeding – If bleeding fails to stop spontaneously give an intravenous infusion of vasopressin 20 units in 200 ml of 5% dextrose over 10–20 min. (This may result in vomiting, defaecation and colic and is contraindicated in patients with ischaemic heart disease).

3. Measures to alleviate the effects of liver failure. (for details see section on "Liver Failure")

4. If bleeding continues despite vasopressin, the use of a Sengst-aken tube should be considered in those patients who are candidates for surgery or injection sclerotherapy of varices. Sengstaken tubes should only be used by those with experience in the procedure as their use is unpleasant for the patient, complex and potentially hazardous.

Liver Biopsy

INDICATIONS

- diagnosis and assessment of cirrhosis
- investigation of hepatomegaly
- investigation of non-obstructive jaundice
- assessment of the treatment of haemachromatosis
- diagnosis of the storage diseases (glycogen storage and amyloid)
- diagnosis of hepatic malignancy
- staging of lymphoma
- granulomatous disease with hepatomegaly.

CONTRAINDICATIONS

- abnormal haemostasis
- infection, including hydatid disease
- ascites and/or severe hepatocellular jaundice

PRECAUTIONS

- the patient must be willing and able to co-operate fully with the procedure.
- haemostasis must be normal: ie. platelets >100,000, APTT and PT normal.
- cross-match 2 units of blood.

LIVER BIOPSY TECHNIQUE

1. Attach Menghini liver biopsy needle, complete with its inner obturating needle, to a 5 ml syringe containing 2 ml of saline. Check patency by ejecting 1 ml of the saline.

2. The position commonly used for liver biopsy is with the patient lying supine with hands folded behind head.

3. Choose the biopsy site, usually intercostal, at the point of maximum dullness in the mid-axillary line, mark chosen point. A subcostal position may be used only if the liver is clearly palpable below the costal margin.

4. Apply a surface antiseptic and drape the field.

5. Practice held expiration; be sure the patient is able to maintain apnoea for 10–15 seconds on instruction.

6. Infiltrate the intercostal space and skin with lignocaine.

7. Make a small skin incision. Never cut through the intercostal muscles.

8. Insert the Menghini needle into the skin incision.

9. Clear the needle by injecting 0.2 ml of saline.

10. Practise the held expiration manouevre again.

11. Pull on syringe as if aspirating. Hold the needle horizontal and at right angles to the patient's body. Order apnoea at the end of normal expiration.

12. Insert the needle in a quick in and out movement as a single step to a depth of 6–8 cm.

13. Gently release the suction on the syringe, then discharge the remaining saline from the syringe to recover the biopsy.

AFTERCARE

– keep the patient in bed for 24 hours after the biopsy.
– pulse rate and blood pressure should be charted frequently (every 30 mins) for 2 hours then, if stable, hourly for 4 hours, continuing 4 hourly for the remainder of the 24 hours.
– examine every few hours for signs of abdominal tenderness suggestive of bleeding.

RISKS AND COMPLICATIONS

– pleurisy and perihepatitis
– haemorrhage
– biliary peritonitis
– puncture of other viscera.

NOTE

It is wise to do a liver biopsy first thing in the morning as the patient is then being monitored at a time at which the most staff are available to recognise and deal with any complications.

Investigation of Jaundice

CLINICAL FEATURES

Pruritis, dark urine, pale stools, pain (suggesting an obstructive cause); weight loss, palpable gallbladder (suggesting malignancy); hepatomegaly, xanthomata and pigmentation in chronic cases.

CAUSES

Pre-hepatic
- haemolysis
- increased red cell turnover.

Intra-hepatic
- viral hepatitis
- cirrhosis
- drug-induced jaundice
- primary biliary cirrhosis
- pericholangitis (inflammatory bowel disease)
- Gilbert's disease

Extra-hepatic
- gallstones
- carcinoma of the pancreas, bile ducts or gallbladder
- secondary carcinoma
- pancreatitis
- bile duct stricture.

INVESTIGATIONS
- FBC, platelets, retics, PT, APTT.
- LFTs (transaminases, alk.phos., proteins, bilirubin).
- anti-mitochondrial and anti-smooth muscle antibodies.
- lipids.
- hepatitis B surface antigen and antibodies.
- protein electrophoresis.
- Isotope scanning can provide evidence of: hepato-splenomegaly, filling defects due to the presence of tumour and occasionally dilated ducts.
- Ultrasound scanning is a rapid, reliable, non-invasive method

of determining whether jaundice is due to extra-hepatic obstruction, by demonstrating the presence of dilated bile ducts when extra-hepatic obstruction is present. It may also demonstrate the presence of stones, secondaries or pancreatic masses.

– Various other techniques exist which may enable specific problems and areas to be investigated, for example:

Liver biopsy can be used to help distinguish between types of intra-hepatic cholestasis once extra-hepatic obstruction has been fully excluded.

Endoscopic retrograde cannulation of the pancreatico-duodenal duct can be used to demonstrate lesions of the pancreas, ampulla and common bileduct.

Thin needle transhepatic cholangiography can deliniate the upper limit of extra-hepatic obstruction. If difficulty is experienced entering the bile ducts it suggests that the jaundice is not due to extra-hepatic obstruction.

SUGGESTED READING

1.   *Medicine* 3rd series 1979 No. 17–18
     Medical Education (International)

2.   Dame Sheila Sherlock
     Diseases of the Liver and Biliary System 6th Ed. 1981
     Blackwell Scientific Publications

6

GASTROENTEROLOGY

ACUTE UPPER GASTROINTESTINAL TRACT HAEMORRHAGE

All patients with a history of haematemesis and/or malaena.

1. Commence i.v. infusion of N saline.
2. Assess circulatory state.

3. Urgent Hb, cross-match 6 units of whole blood
4. Keep patient nil by mouth
5. When convenient check platelets, PT, blood urea

NOT SHOCKED

Correct anaemia if present

Arrange gastroscopy

Cimetidine 200 mg i.v. q.d.s.
(value uncertain)

Antacids p.r.n.

CONDITION STABLE
Start oral fluids

SHOCKED

Resuscitate rapidly with FFP
and blood as soon as arrives
(O-ve if sufficiently urgent)
CVP line advisable
Contact a Surgeon
Continue rapid transfusion until:
(a) pulse <90/min
(b) systolic B.P. >100 mmHg
(c) CVP stabilised
(d) urine output >50 ml/hr

CONDITION STABLE
Gastroscope
Cimetidine 200 mg i.v. q.d.s.

Start oral fluids

In the event of failure
to stabilise or rebleeding
contact the surgeons.

Peptic Ulceration

The classical symptoms of peptic ulceration are well known but are frequently not present, and are not specific enough for a definite diagnosis to be made. If the symptoms are sufficiently severe to warrant specific treatment, i.e. drugs with ulcer healing properties rather than antacids, the diagnosis must be confirmed on either gastroscopy or barium meal before treatment is commenced.

DUODENAL ULCER

- stop: smoking, excess alcohol intake, ulcerogenic drugs (eg. aspirin or other NSAIDs)
- normal diet
- cimetidine 200 mg t.d.s. and 400 mg nocte for 6 weeks
- antacids p.r.n.

The symptoms of a duodenal ulcer normally improve rapidly on treatment with cimetidine. If the symptoms persist check for possible aggravating factors again and arrange repeat endoscopy to assess healing. In event of failure to heal replace cimetidine with:

- ranitidine 150 mg b.d. (for 1 month)

or - bismuth chelate 5 ml q.d.s.

or - carbenoxolone 50 mg q.d.s. (in younger patients only and monitor potassium and BP).

Patients failing to respond to standard treatment should be investigated further to exclude the presence of underlying conditions such as Zollinger-Ellison syndrome.

Indications for surgical treatment of duodenal ulceration

- failed medical treatment
- excessive time off work
- frequent relapses
- complications such as perforation, haemorrhage or obstruction.

GASTRIC ULCERATION

If the diagnosis has been made on barium meal, arrangements should be made for endoscopy and biopsy to be performed.

Give medical treatment as for duodenal ulceration and continue for 6 weeks. At the end of this period the patient should be re-endoscoped and a biopsy performed if the lesion has not healed because of the risk of malignancy.

Indications for surgery of gastric ulcer
- as for duodenal ulcer plus
- resection of possible or definite malignancy.

GASTRO-OESOPHAGEAL REFLUX AND OESOPHAGITIS

The diagnosis of these conditions is based on a history of: retrosternal pain (particularly associated with lying flat or bending forward), acid reflux and flatulence. Confirmation of the diagnosis may be made by barium studies or endoscopy.

Management
- reduce reflux by avoiding stooping and sleeping with the head of the bed raised by approximately 10 cm on blocks
- stop smoking – reduce weight – antacids
- cimetidine 200 mg t.d.s. and 400 mg nocte – metoclopramide 10 mg t.d.s.

Ulcerative Colitis

Symptoms include diarrhoea with blood and mucus mixed with the stool, abdominal distension and discomfort relieved by defaecation, and tenesmus. In severe cases fever, sweating and weight loss occur.

Investigations

- FBC, ESR.
- U+E, LFTs.
- stool for pathogens.
- sigmoidoscopy and biopsy ⎫
⎬ with great care in patients with severe attacks due to
- barium enema ⎭ risk of perforation.

ROUTINE MANAGEMENT

- high fibre diet
- iron supplements as required
- sulphasalazine 500 mg t.d.s.

MILD/MODERATE ATTACKS

- in these attacks the patient remains systemically well but is

passing frequent motions eg. 6 to 8 daily
- routine management as above

plus
- steroid enema daily
- a short course of prednisolone commencing with 5 mg q.d.s., continuing until symptoms settle then reducing rapidly.

SEVERE ATTACKS
- the patient is systemically ill with: fever, anorexia and weight loss and has a serious and potentially lethal condition.
- watch carefully for signs of acute dilatation suggested by pain (may be absent due to high dose steroids), distension, increase in pulse rate, and fall in blood pressure. If suspicious arrange urgent plain X-ray of abdomen.
- intravenous fluids to correct dehydration.
- blood transfusion if anaemic.
- hydrocortisone 100 mg i.v. q.d.s. changing to reducing dose of oral prednisolone when condition settling.
- parenteral feeding (discuss with dietician).

Crohn's Disease

The basic principles are very similar to those for treatment of ulcerative colitis including:
- general supportive measures: iron supplements, blood, and intravenous fluids as required.
- sulphasalazine maintenance treatment.
- corticosteroids during acute attacks.

Malabsorption

SYMPTOMS AND SIGNS OF MALABSORPTION
- diarrhoea
- abdominal distension
- weight loss
- steatorrhoea (pale, frequent, loose, foul-smelling motions which float and are difficult to flush away).
- symptoms and signs of secondary deficiencies: anaemia, bone pain, glossitis, dermatitis, bruising, weakness.
  A history of previous gastric or bowel surgery may obviously be of importance.

INVESTIGATIONS

- FBC and ESR.
- U+E, LFTs.
- calcium, phosphate, alkaline phosphatase.
- serum proteins
- iron, total iron binding capacity.
- B_{12} and folate.
- examination of the stool for ova and parasites.
- 3 day faecal fat excretion.
- xylose absorption test. D-xylose is a relatively inert sugar which is absorbed but only minimally metabolised, then excreted by the kidney. 5 g of xylose is given by mouth and the urine collected for 5 hours. The excretion of <1.2 g of xylose is abnormal.
- ^{14}C-glycocholate breath test. In the presence of small bowel overgrowth the ^{14}C-labelled glycocholate is broken down by the bacteria and the ^{14}C is released to be detected as CO_2 in the breath.
- Small bowel radiology (barium follow-through). Abnormal signs include loss of the feathery pattern of the mucosa, distension of the lumen, increased flocculation of the barium, blind loops, diverticuli, fistuli and the "string" sign (Crohn's disease).
- Small bowel biopsy. Findings include total villous atrophy in coeliac disease, partial villous atrophy, lymphoma, amyloid, absent disaccharidase activity, and Whipple's disease.

INVESTIGATIONS OF THE PANCREAS

- plain abdominal X-ray for calcification
- ultrasound scanning
- endoscopic retrograde cannulation of the pancreatico - duodenal duct allows visualisation of the pancreatic and common bile ducts
- pancreatic function tests (difficult and unsatisfactory)

Acute Pancreatitis

CLINICAL FEATURES

Mild attack – abdominal pain, nausea and vomiting and a mild degree of shock (tachycardia, systolic BP 80–100 mmHg)

Severe attack – severe shock, persistent severe abdominal pain with guarding and rigidity, prolonged vomiting, paralytic ileus, pleural effusion and "shock" lung, ecchymoses over the flanks or periumbilical areas, indicating retroperitoneal haemorrhage in haemorrhagic pancreatitis.

Severe episodes of pancreatitis have a considerable mortality rate (25%+)

CAUSES

- gallstones
- alcohol
- hypercalcaemia
- hyperlipidaemia
- viral infections
- drugs: steroids, phenothiazines, oral contraceptives, thiazides.
- hypothermia.

INVESTIGATIONS

- FBC, platelets, and blood film. (look for evidence of DIC).
- U+E, LFTs, blood glucose.
- calcium (hypocalcaemia is almost invariably present).
- serum amylase: a very high level (>1000 units) is strongly suggestive of acute pancreatitis, moderate elevations can occur in perforated duodenal ulcer amongst other conditions. A normal level does not firmly exclude the diagnosis as acute haemorrhagic pancreatitis has been reported in the presence of a normal amylase.
- chest X-ray
- plain abdominal X-ray (erect and supine), may show evidence of gas under the diaphragm in a perforated DU, one of the main differential diagnoses. The typical appearance in pancreatitis is the 'sentinal loop', a dilated loop of small bowel overlying the pancreas.
- ultrasound is useful in the diagnosis of acute pancreatitis, the typical appearance being an enlarged pancreas. Ultrasound may also demonstrate gallstones which are still the most common cause of pancreatitis in this country.

TREATMENT

1. Treatment of shock with
    – intravenous fluids
    – plasma
    – whole blood.

2. Pain relief with pethidine 50–100 mg i.m. (other opiates are contraindicated).

3. Nasogastric tube.

4. Correct the metabolic problems which may occur;
    hyperglycaemia – insulin (small doses only are required)
    hypocalcaemia – calcium gluconate 10 ml of a 10% solution either as intermittent i.v. injections or added to i.v. fluids. Repeat depending on the response.

5. "Specific" treatments such as glucagon or aprotinin have NOT proved to be effective.

6. Antibiotics are only indicated if there is evidence of infection.

7. Surgery. If in doubt about the diagnosis refer for laparotomy to look for a surgically correctable lesion. If the patient has pancreatitis the laparotomy increases the mortality.

SUGGESTED FURTHER READING

1. *Medicine* third series nos. 14–17 1979
    Medical Education (International)

2. M.W. Dronfield, M.J.S. Langman
    Acute Upper Gastro-intestinal Tract Bleeding.
    British Journal of Hospital Medicine 1978 19:97

7

RENAL MEDICINE

Renal Failure

PRE-RENAL RENAL FAILURE

Functional renal insufficiency due to pre-renal causes such as:
- hypovolaemia and hypotension from haemorrhage, burns, fluid loss.
- septicaemic shock.
- poor cardiac output

Diagnosis of pre-renal failure.
- urine specific gravity > 1020
- urine/plasma urea ratio > 10
- urine/plasma osmolality ratio >2
- urine sodium <20 mmol/l.

If the cause is severe and prolonged then acute tubular necrosis may occur.

INTRINSIC RENAL FAILURE

Acute
- acute tubular necrosis
- acute glomerulonephritis
- acute interstitial nephritis.

Chronic
- chronic glomerulonephritis
- hypertension
- chronic pyelonephritis
- congenital eg.polycystic kidneys
- analgesic nephropathy.

Diagnosis of intrinsic renal failure.
   urine specific gravity <1020
   urine/plasma urea ratio <10
   urine/plasma osmolality ratio <1.2
   urine sodium >70 mmol/l.

POST-RENAL RENAL FAILURE

Acute
   – bilateral calculi
   – precipitation of urate
   – damage to ureters.
Chronic
   – prostatic hypertrophy
   – renal calculi
   – retro-peritoneal fibrosis.
Features suggestive of post-renal renal failure include
   – complete anuria
   – large prostate
   – large bladder
   – calculi
   – large kidneys on X-ray or ultrasound
   – normal urine sediment on microscopy

INVESTIGATION OF RENAL FAILURE

The history should include details of drug intake, with particular reference to potentially nephrotoxic drugs such as analgesics (over prolonged periods), cephaloridine, aminoglycosides, sulphonamides, gold or penicillamine. Also check for a history of exposure to nephrotoxic substances including organic solvents and heavy metals. Clinical examination should include close scrutiny for evidence of other systemic diseases such as diabetes, hypertension or SLE.

Routine Investigations
Blood
   FBC, reticulocyte count, platelets, blood film
   – U+E, creatinine
   – osmolality
   – calcium, phosphate, alkaline phosphatase
   – blood sugar

- hepatitis associated antigens
- blood gases

Urine

- culture
- microscopy
- Labstix for blood and protein
- 24 hour collection for U+E, creatinine and protein
- osmolality

Ward

- daily weight
- input/output chart
- BP chart
- temperature chart

General Investigations

- chest X-ray (for cardiac size, pulmonary oedema, infection, etc.)
- plain abdominal X-ray (for renal size)
- ECG
- Ultrasound for renal size and calculi

Definitive Investigations

1. IVP (high dose infusion required when blood urea >15 mmol/l).
   small kidneys – no further investigations required.
   normal sized kidneys – procede to renal biopsy.
   large kidneys – investigate for possible obstruction.

2. Cystoscopy and retrograde pyelograms if obstruction is suspected.

3. Renal biopsy.

MANAGEMENT OF PRE-RENAL FAILURE

Before acute tubular necrosis becomes established it is often possible to reverse the oliguria.

1. Rapid correction of hypovolaemia (when giving i.v. infusions avoid forearm veins as these may be required for fistulae in the future. Veins on the dorsum of the hand or in the cubital fossa should be used).

2. Treatment of septicaemia.

3. Mannitol; 200 ml of a 20% solution by i.v. infusion over 30 min OR frusemide 100 mg by slow i.v. injection. If no increase in urine output is achieved within 60 min repeat with 250 mg by i.v. infusion over 20 min. If there is no response to the diuretics, the patient should then be treated as having established renal failure.

MANAGEMENT OF ESTABLISHED RENAL FAILURE

General Measures such as the removal of exacerbating factors including:
   - Infection, systemic or urinary tract.
   - Potentially nephrotoxic drugs.
   - Severe hypertension.
   - Avoid the use of a urinary catheter.

Hydration
This can be judged roughly by clinical methods such as skin turgor and JVP, and accurately by the use of a CVP line (see "Monitoring Central Venous Pressure"). If fluid depletion is suggested by clinical methods or by a low CVP give N saline i.v. infusion 500 ml hourly and review the clinical response and CVP at least hourly.

If the patient is normally hydrated the fluid requirements are the volume of the previous 24 hours urine output and any losses from fistulae etc. plus 500 ml. If overhydration is a problem, which it commonly is, fluids should be restricted further until a fall in weight is achieved.

Monitoring of fluid balance obviously requires carefully kept input and output charts and, more important, accurate daily weight charts. If there appears to be a discrepancy between fluid charts and weight charts use the latter to guide fluid intake, reducing fluid intake if weight is increasing. If a patient is severely overhydrated peritoneal dialysis may be required to correct or prevent the ensuing complications especially pulmonary oedema.

Electrolyte Balance

1. Potassium – hyperkalaemia. If the serum potassium is >7.0 mmol/l there is a significant danger of cardiac arrest. If the typical ECG changes of hyperkalaemia are present (see ECG - electrolyte changes) then rapid treatment is required. If not then

treatment can procede at a slower rate as the risk of arrhythmias is smaller.

Rapid treatment of hyperkalaemia
- calcium gluconate, 10 ml of a 10% solution as a slow i.v. injection, reduces the cardiotoxic effects of the hyperkalaemia.
- followed by 100 ml of 50% dextrose containing 20 units of soluble insulin.

This buys sufficient time for more definitive treatment, such as peritoneal dialysis, to be set up.

Slow treatment – calcium resonium 15 g 2–4 times daily orally or 30 g as an enema.

Long-term treatment – a low potassium diet (40 mmol/day) and avoidance of potassium containing drugs.

Hypokalaemia – this is often an advantage in the early stages if not too severe (>2.8 mmol/l)

2.   Sodium – Restrict sodium intake to a diet with no added salt if fluid overload or hypertension is present. Changes in serum sodium reflect changes in fluid status rather than body sodium. Sodium lost through diarrhoea, nasogastric tube drainage or excessive loss in the urine in sodium-losing nephropathy or in the diuretic phase after removal of an obstructive lesion, should be replaced.

3.   Phosphate – Hyperphosphataemia should be controlled at an early stage to retard the development of renal osteodystrophy. Reduce dietary intake as a first step then add aluminium hydroxide 10 mls t.d.s. increasing to 30 ml t.d.s. if dietary measures alone fail to control the hyperphosphataemia. Aluminium toxicity is a potential hazard of longterm treatment and must be considered particularly if any neurological symptoms develop.

4.   Hypocalcaemia – Control the hyperphosphataemia which will inevitably be present then add calcium supplements if a raised serum alkaline phosphate suggests progressive bone disease. In a few cases 1-alpha-hydroxycholecalciferol 1 microgram daily may be required to control bone disease.

Nutrition
Restrict protein intake to 40 g per day of high biological value

protein, in consultation with the dietician. When on haemodialysis, 60–80 g per day are normally allowed; no restriction of protein intake is required when on peritoneal dialysis. A high carbohydrate and fat intake is required providing 30–50 calories/kg to produce a protein-sparing effect. Additional kilojoules can be provided in the form of high carbohydrate low electrolyte drinks such as Hycal or Caloreen. Vitamin supplements and folic acid 5 mg daily are advisable and, in patients on haemodialysis, iron supplements to compensate for blood loss.

Drugs

Many drugs are excreted by the kidney and should be used in reduced dosage or avoided in patients with renal failure. For an extensive list of drugs and appropriate modifications to dosage see British National Formulary.

Recommended drugs for common problems include:

Nausea, vomiting
- metoclopramide 5 mg oral or i.m.

Pain
- paracetamol 1 g, but avoid in severe renal failure.
- morphine or diamorphine in reduced dosage eg 2.5 mg i.m.

Anticonvulsants
- diazepam.
- phenytoin; start at 200 mg daily then check level and adjust if necessary.

Sedation
- diazepam

Diuretics
- frusemide; initially in a dose of 40–80 mg, double dose until desired effect is achieved. In emergency give 250 mg by i.v. infusion over 20 min (rapid i.v. injection risks ototoxicity).

Antibiotics
- benzylpenicillin maximum dose 6 mega units daily.
- ampicillin max. dose 250 mg t.d.s.
- trimethoprim 100–200 mg daily.
- gentamicin, initially 80 mg i.m. daily adjusting dose depending on blood levels.

Antihypertensives
- propranolol, starting in low dosage, 20 mg t.d.s. or atenolol 50 mg daily.
- hydralazine, 25 mg b.d. initially then increase.

INDICATIONS FOR PERITONEAL DIALYSIS

- hyperkalaemia failing to respond to conservative treatment
- fluid overload
- symptoms i.e. nausea, vomiting, drowsiness, fits or pericarditis
- rapidly rising blood urea (>16 mmol daily)
- blood urea >33 mmol/l in acute renal failure.

RELATIVE CONTRAINDICATIONS TO PERITONEAL DIALYSIS

- recent abdominal surgery
- peritoneal drains, adhesions or fistulae
- respiratory insufficiency
- diabetes mellitus.

Renal Biopsy

Indications
- nephrotic syndrome
- renal failure in a patient with normal sized kidneys
- investigation of proteinuria (which see)
- to judge the response of parenchymal disease to treatment
- investigation of haematuria with normal IVP.

Preparation of a patient prior to renal biopsy
- must have normal PT, APTT, and platelet count.
- 2 units of blood cross-matched.
- IVP showing both kidneys functioning.
- control hypertension so that the diastolic blood pressure is <100 mmHg.
- if the patient is uraemic or oliguric, dialyse before biopsy to reduce the risk of bleeding.

POST BIOPSY CARE

- keep the patient in bed for 24 hours.
- frequent pulse and BP recordings (1/2 hourly initially).
- microscopic haematuria occurs in almost all cases.
- macroscopic haematuria occurs in a minority of cases and may lead to episodes of clot colic.
- abdominal pain and discomfort need to be watched carefully as they may indicate significant renal bleeding.

Investigation of Proteinuria

ROUTINE URINE TESTING FOR PROTEIN
(Albustix +ve >40 mg/l, normal urine <20 mg/l)

HISTORY AND EXAMINATION

FIRST LINE INVESTIGATIONS   urine - culture and microscopy
- 24 hour sample for protein
- sample for protein after rest
blood - U+E creatinine
- glucose

TRANSIENT OR ORTHOSTATIC	→	IF OTHERWISE NORMAL DISCHARGE	INCIDENTAL CAUSES
			- fever
			- severe exertion
			- cold exposure
			- abdo.operations
			- transfusions

SECOND LINE INVESTIGATIONS   - IVP
- ANF
- protein electrophoresis

→ <2 g PROTEIN DAILY ———→ FOLLOW

>2 g PROTEIN DAILY ————————

ABNORMAL FIRST LINE   EVIDENCE OF
INVESTIGATIONS   MULTISYSTEM DISEASE

→ RENAL BIOPSY ←

Investigation of Haematuria

CAUSES

1. Renal – glomerulonephritis, polycystic disease, calculi, tumours, TB, analgesic nephropathy.

2. Lower renal tract – calculi, tumours, prostatic hypertrophy.

3. Miscellaneous – bleeding disorders and anticoagulants.

INVESTIGATIONS

- urine microscopy and culture
- urine protein and sugar
- urine cytology
- U+E
- FBC and platelets
- IVP
- cystoscopy (when IVP and culture are normal)
- red cells and protein in the urine suggest a glomerular origin and are indications for renal biopsy.

SUGGESTED READING

1. Roger Gabriel
   Postgraduate Nephrology 2nd Ed. 1978
   Butterworths

2. Sir Douglas Black and N.F. Jones
   Renal Disease 4th Ed. 1979
   Blackwell Scientific Publications

8

ENDOCRINOLOGY AND METABOLISM

Thyrotoxicosis

COMMON CAUSES

– Graves' disease (hyperplasia)
– toxic nodular goitre.

CLINICAL FEATURES

Include: weight loss, tachycardia, arrhythmias, tremor, weakness, diarrrhoea, lid-lag, lid retraction, goitre etc. Particularly in older patients the signs may be much less dramatic with weight loss, heart failure and atrial fibrillation being the only features.

INVESTIGATIONS

– FBC
– U+E, serum calcium
– T_4, T_3 uptake, FTI
– TRH test if FTI borderline
– T_3 (in a patient with normal T_4 but the clinical picture of hyperthyroidism)
– ECG
– chest X-ray (looking for retrosternal goitre, evidence of cardiac failure).

MANAGEMENT

Medical
– short term reduction of sympathetic effects by propranolol 40 mg t.d.s., increasing if necessary. Continue for 4–6 weeks until

anti-thyroid drugs take effect.
- long term reduction of thyroid activity by carbimazole, 10 mg t.d.s. for 4–6 weeks, which normally controls the hyperthyroidism.
- once the hyperthyroidism has been controlled clinically and biochemically, change to a maintenance dose of carbimazole of 5 mg t.d.s., reducing further depending on the results of the thyroid function tests.
- occasionally a higher dose of carbimazole, up to 60 mg daily, is required to produce control.
- continue the carbimazole for 12 months, then stop and observe. Approximately 50% of patients will relapse; they should again be controlled on carbimazole before being considered for treatment with radio-iodine or surgery.

Radioactive Iodine Treatment
Indications
- failed drug treatment in men over 40 years of age and postmenopausal women.
- patients unable to take or tolerate oral medication.
- for elderly patients who are unfit for surgery.

Disadvantages
- patients treated with radioactive iodine must be followed for life as there is a high incidence of late hypothyroidism. Some units have attempted to overcome this by giving ablative doses of ^{131}I and starting all patients on lifelong replacement thyroxine.

Surgery
Indications
- failed medical treatment in young people.
- patients with large goitres.

Patients must be rendered euthyroid before surgery can take place.

THYROID CRISIS

This is a rare complication of severe untreated hyperthyroidism and is provoked by stress such as infection or surgery. The symptoms and signs are those of hyperthyroidism plus extreme anxiety, hyperpyrexia and left ventricular failure.

Treatment
- propranolol 40 mg t.d.s.
- carbimazole 20 mg t.d.s.

– Lugol's solution (iodine solution) 0.5ml t.d.s. Delay for at least 2 hours after the carbimazole has been given.
– correction of fluid and electrolyte balance.
– treatment of cardiac failure if present.

Myxoedema

CLINICAL FEATURES

Fatigue, physical and mental slowness, weight increase, gruff voice, dry skin and hair, carpal tunnel syndrome and cerebellar signs, menorrhagia, deafness, and psychosis.

INVESTIGATIONS

– FBC (frequently anaemic, may be micro-, normo-, or macrocytic)
– ECG (may show low voltage, flat T waves, long QT interval, sinus bradycardia and AV block)
– chest X-ray
– thyroid antibodies
– T_4, T_3 uptake, and TSH.

MANAGEMENT

– commence thyroxine in small doses, 50 μg daily.
– in patients with ischaemic heart disease, reduce dose to 25 μg daily
– increase the dose by 50 μg every 4 weeks until maintenance dose is reached, usually 100–300 μg daily.
– adequacy of maintenance dose is judged by FTI and TSH levels returning to normal.

MYXOEDEMA COMA

This is a rare complication of myxoedema, and requires large doses of thyroxine (400–500 μg) by nasogastric tube or intravenously. Assess associated hypoadrenalism and hypothermia.

Addison's Disease

CLINICAL FEATURES

Include pigmentation of the skin and mucosae, lassitude and muscle weakness, postural hypotension, weight loss, nausea, abdominal pain, vitiligo, and hypoglycaemia.

CAUSES

- autoimmune adrenalitis
- tuberculosis
- metastatic carcinoma
- amyloid
- haemochromatosis
- haemorrhage into the adrenals (meningococcal septicaemia and DIC)

INVESTIGATIONS

- U+E and blood glucose (typically $\downarrow$ Na, $\uparrow$ K, $\uparrow$ urea, $\downarrow$ blood glucose).
- plasma cortisol (may be within the normal range but this is inappropriate for a patient under the stress of illness when high levels are expected).
- anti-adrenal antibodies.
- chest X-ray for evidence of TB.
- plain abdominal X-ray for evidence of adrenal calcification suggesting a tuberculous etiology.

If the patient is obviously unwell and requires treatment with steroids before the Synacthen test can take place, use dexamethasone as the steroid replacement as it does not interfere significantly with the plasma cortisol levels measured during the Synacthen test.

Short Synacthen test. Take baseline plasma cortisol, preferably at 9am. Give Synacthen 250 μg i.m. then take blood for plasma cortisol at 30 and 60 min. Normally the basal cortisol should excede 170 nmol/l, and should rise to a peak value >600 nmol/l, with an increment of >190 nmol/l.

If the short Synacthen test is abnormal or equivocal a long Synacthen test should be performed.

Long Synacthen test. Take blood for basal plasma cortisol at 9am, give Synacthen depot 1 mg i.m. Take blood samples for cortisol at 1,4,8, and 24 hours. In patients with Addison's disease the response is impaired and the plasma cortisol does not excede 600 nmol/l. In patients with hypopituitarism a delayed response occurs.

MANAGEMENT

Acute Hypoadrenalism
- give 100 mg hydrocortisone i.v.
- continue 100 mg hydrocortisone i.m. q.d.s.
- erect an i.v. line and infuse 1 l of N.saline in 1 hour.
- if hypoglycaemia is present use N.saline in 5% dextrose.
- continue N.saline so that 4–6 l are given in 24 hours.
- change to oral hydrocortisone after 24 hours, reducing the dosage to a maintenance dose of 20–30 mg of hydrocortisone in 2 doses, and add fludrocortisone 50–200 μg daily.

Chronic Hypoadrenalism
- commence maintenance dose of hydrocortisone 10 mg b.d. orally increasing to a total of 30 mg daily if required. If 30 mg are required give as 20 mg a.m. and 10 mg p.m.
- add fludrocortisone 50–200 μg daily depending on requirements to maintain normal blood pressure, particularly standing blood pressure, and eliminate postural hypotension.
- increase the dose if fatigue, hypotension, raised plasma urea or potassium occur.
- increase the dose if the patient is unwell for any reason. Allow the patient to double the normal dose temporarily without seeking advice.

Management of Patients on Long Term Steroids Over Periods of Stress

Minor Surgery
- hydrocortisone 100 mg q.d.s. for 48 hours, commencing 2 hours prior to surgery (give with pre-med).
- after 48 hours change back to normal maintenance dose.
- fludrocortisone is not required until the dose of hydrocortisone is reduced below 60 mg daily.

Major Surgery
- hydrocortisone 100 mg q.d.s. i.m. for 3–5 days.
- change to oral doses, and gradually reduce the dosage until it is back to maintenance dose after a further 3–4 days.
- if the patient remains unwell or develops complications

reintroduce the full i.m. dosage.
– fludrocortisone is not required until the dose of hydrocortisone falls below 60 mg daily.

Other Stress

eg. myocardial infarction or trauma, treat as for major surgery.

For patients on steroids in therapeutic doses rather than as replacement treatment treat as above, unless already on large doses (>30 mg prednisolone daily), when this is likely to prove sufficient as long as absorption can be guaranteed. If in doubt change to i.m. hydrocortisone.

Electrolyte Disturbances

CAUSES OF HYPERNATRAEMIA

1. Water loss in excess of sodium loss
        – gastroenteritis
        – unconscious/confused patient
        – osmotic diuresis (diabetic comas).

2. Excess sodium replacement
        – i.v. saline
        – increased oral intake.

3. Sodium retention
        – primary hyperaldosteronism
        – corticosteroids and Cushing's syndrome.

4. Failure of water retention
        – pituitary diabetes insipidus
        – nephrogenic diabetes insipidus
            hereditary
            partial obstruction
            myeloma
            hypercalcaemia
            hypokalaemia

CAUSES OF HYPONATRAEMIA

1. Sodium loss in excess of water
        – prolonged vomiting
        – severe diarrhoea
        – small gut fistulae
        – excessive sweating

2. Failure of renal sodium retention
    – Addison's disease
    – sodium losing nephritis
        chronic pyelonephritis
        analgesic nephropathy
        relief of obstruction
    – diabetic ketoacidosis
    – excess diuretics

3. Excess water
    – i.v. replacement
    – compulsive water drinking
    – inappropriate ADH secretion
        malignant tumours particularly oat cell carcinomas
        head injury
        lung disease
        acute porphyria

CAUSES OF HYPERKALAEMIA

1. Failure of renal excretion
    – reduced sodium/potassium exchange : hypoadrenalism
    – reduced exchangable sodium :
        renal failure
        sodium depletion
        potassium-sparing diuretics.

2. Increased extracellular fluid potassium
    – anoxia
    – acidosis
    – diabetic ketoacidosis
    – severe tissue damage
    – severe starvation.

Treatment of Hyperkalaemia
    – see under "Renal Failure"

CAUSES OF HYPOKALAEMIA

1. Renal loss
    – diuretics (thiazide and loop)
    – excess corticosteroids
        therapeutic

Cushing's syndrome and disease
- primary hyperaldosteronism
- secondary hyperaldosteronism
    heart failure
    cirrhosis
    severe hypertension
- uncontrolled diabetes mellitus (particularly during treatment).
- ingestion of carbenoxolone or liquorice derivitives
- distal tubular disease
  renal tubular acidosis
  Fanconi's syndrome.

2. Gastro-intestinal loss
    - prolonged vomiting
    - diarrhoea
    - fistulae
    - prolonged gastric aspiration
    - purgative abuse
    - ureteric drainage into the bowel
    - mucus secreting tumours.

3. Insufficient intake
   - malabsorption
   - diet.

SEVERE HYPERCALCAEMIA

Symptoms include thirst, polyuria, polydipsia, weakness, constipation and mental confusion. Severe hypercalcaemia can cause fatal arrhythmias, coma or acute renal failure. If symptomatic, the serum calcium level is normally >3.5 mmol/l.

Causes
   - metastatic malignancy
   - non-metastatic manifestation of malignancy (tumour producing PTH or similar product)
   - hyperparathyroidism
   - myeloma
   - vitamin D toxicity
   - sarcoidosis.

Investigations
- U+E, calcium (ionised and total), phosphate, alkaline phosphatase
- protein electrophoresis
- X-rays of chest and hands.

Management
1. Patients with severe hypercalcaemia are always dehydrated. Rehydration and saline diuresis are important steps in management. A CVP line is useful in monitoring treatment particularly in those patients with cardiovascular problems.

2. Give N saline 1 l in 2 hours, then 1 l every 4 hours, with potassium supplements as required.

3. Once dehydration has been corrected (after 4–6 l), give frusemide 40 mg with each litre of saline, increasing to maintain the diuresis. Rehydration and saline diuresis frequently produce a satisfactory reduction in hypercalcaemia.

4. Calcitonin 4–8 units/kg daily i.m. is a useful adjunct to rehydration particularly in patients with malignant disease.

5. Prednisolone 30 mg daily produces a slow reduction in serum calcium level in some patients with malignant disease. A significant reduction is not achieved before 7–10 days.

6. Mithramycin 15 μg/kg daily is an effective drug in the control of hypercalcaemia. Its toxicity restricts its use to patients not responding to other drugs.

Diabetes Mellitus

CLASSIFICATION OF DIABETES MELLITUS
It is possible to classify diabetes mellitus into four classes.

Insulin Dependent Diabetes Mellitus (IDDM)
This is characterised by decreased production of insulin, with a body mass which is usually normal or decreased. Ketoacidosis results if it is untreated. It tends to occur in children, adolescents and young adults.

Non Insulin Dependent Diabetes Mellitus (NIDDM)
Characterised by increasing frequency with age, usually increased

body mass, normal or increased endogenous insulin production (but not as high as would be expected from a normal person exposed to the same level of hyperglycaemia), a tendency to develop hyperglycaemia but not ketoacidosis.

Gestational Diabetes Mellitus (GDM)

The appearance of diabetes during pregnancy with remission after delivery.

Impaired Glucose Tolerance

This is diagnosed on the basis of blood glucose levels during a GTT (for levels see below)

DIAGNOSTIC BLOOD GLUCOSE CONCENTRATIONS

Diabetes mellitus
- fasting blood glucose > 7 mmol/l
- random blood glucose > 11 mmol/l
- glucose tolerance test: fasting > 7 mmol/l, 2 hour > 11 mmol/l.

Impaired glucose tolerance
- fasting blood glucose < 7 mmol/l
- GTT 2 hour blood glucose > 8 mmol/l, < 11 mmol/l.

Causes of diabetes mellitus include:
- endocrine causes: acromegaly, Cushing's syndrome
- drugs: corticosteroids, thiazide diuretics
- metabolic causes: haemochromatosis
- miscellaneous: pancreatitis, cystic fibrosis.

CHECKLIST FOR CONTROL OF DIABETES

1. symptoms – polyuria, thirst, polydipsia.

2. hypoglycaemic attacks.

3. ketoacidosis.

4. blood glucose, and glycosylated haemoglobin levels.

5. urine testing – glycosuria, ketonuria, protein.

6. weight.

7. fundi.

8. feet and skin infections.

DIABETIC COMPLICATIONS

At regular intervals diabetic complications should be assessed.
1. Specific complications due to glycosylation of basement membrane proteins.

(a) retinopathy and cataracts
     – visual acuity, and opthalmoscopy.
     – slit lamp examination, and fluorescein angiography to confirm retinopathy in difficult cases.
     – referral for laser coagulation if new vessel formation seen.

(b) nephropathy
     – urine testing for protein.
     – serum creatinine.

(c) neuropathy
     – sensation (including vibration sensation)
     – reflexes
     – autonomic neuropathy.

2. Non-specific complications
   (a) hyperlipidaemia.
   (b) macroangiopathy – peripheral pulses and ECG.
   (c) infective complications.

ORAL ANTI-DIABETIC AGENTS

Function – to supplement the effects of diet, NOT to replace diet.

1. Sulphonylureas
   action – stimulation of Beta cells
   short acting – tolbutamide 0.5–2.0 g daily in divided doses.
   medium acting – glibenclamide 2.5–15 mg daily in single a.m. dose
   long acting – chlorpropamide 100–300 mg daily in single a.m. dose.

2. Biguanides
   actions
   – only work in the presence of functioning Beta cells.
   – reduce glucose absorption from the gut.
   – reduce glucose oxidation.
   Metformin 0.5–1.7 g daily in divided doses.
   Contraindicated in renal and liver impairment.

ROUTINE MANAGEMENT OF DIABETES MELLITUS

Diet

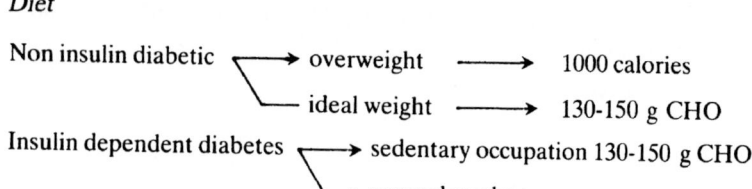

INSULIN PREPARATIONS

	Onset	*Peak*	*Duration*
SHORT – ACTING			
SOLUBLE INSULIN	30 min	2-4 hours	6-8 hours
ACTRAPID	30 min	2-5 hours	6-8 hours
INTERMEDIATE – ACTING			
ISOPHANE	2 hours	5-12 hours	18 hours
INSULATARD	2 hours	4-12 hours	24 hours
LONG – ACTING			
LENTE	3 hours	6-14 hours	22-30 hours
MONOTARD	3 hours	6-14 hours	22 hours

Management of Diabetic Emergencies

HYPOGLYCAEMIA

Typical clinical signs include: sweating, pallor. dilated pupils, and tachycardia. Suspect in any diabetic patient who is confused, drowsy or appears to have had a stroke. Alcohol may be responsible for provoking the hypoglycaemia.

- Take blood for glucose level and Dextrostix test (use fresh Dextrostix, preferably foil packed, as older samples are unreliable) or B.M. 20–800 stick.
- If conscious give oral glucose.
- If unconscious inject 40 ml of 50% dextrose i.v. and repeat if necessary.

FLOW CHART OF MANAGEMENT

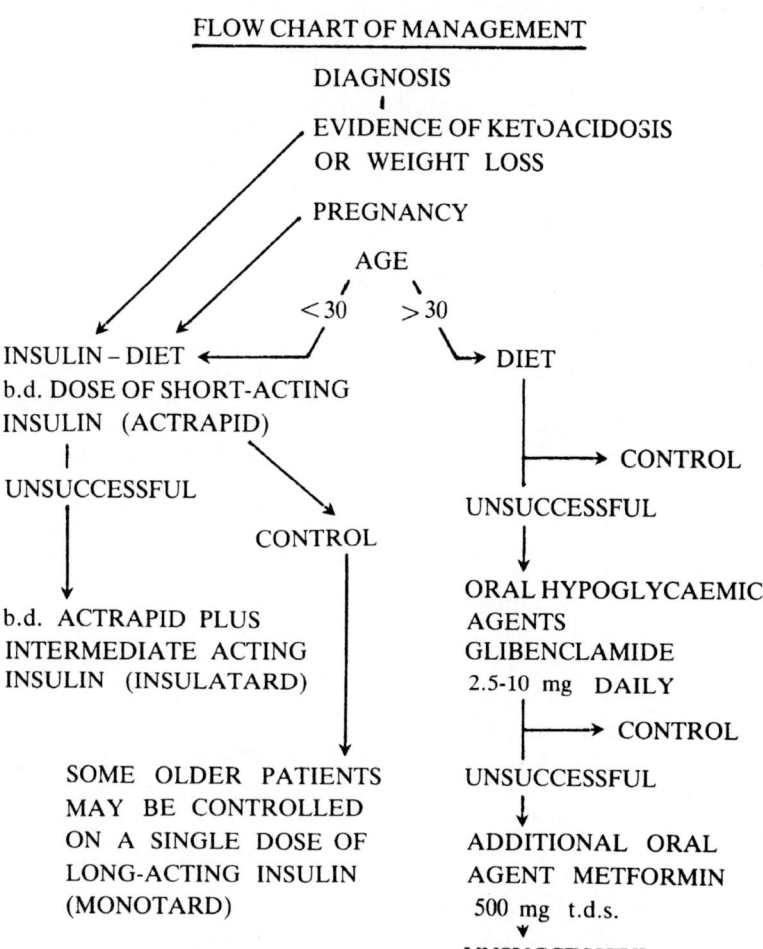

DIAGNOSIS

EVIDENCE OF KETOACIDOSIS OR WEIGHT LOSS

PREGNANCY

AGE

<30   >30

INSULIN – DIET   ←   → DIET
b.d. DOSE OF SHORT-ACTING
INSULIN (ACTRAPID)
                                    → CONTROL

UNSUCCESSFUL   UNSUCCESSFUL

            CONTROL   ORAL HYPOGLYCAEMIC
                            AGENTS
b.d. ACTRAPID PLUS   GLIBENCLAMIDE
INTERMEDIATE ACTING   2.5-10 mg DAILY
INSULIN (INSULATARD)
                                    → CONTROL

                            UNSUCCESSFUL
SOME OLDER PATIENTS
MAY BE CONTROLLED   ADDITIONAL ORAL
ON A SINGLE DOSE OF   AGENT METFORMIN
LONG-ACTING INSULIN   500 mg t.d.s.
(MONOTARD)
                            UNSUCCESSFUL

                            INSULIN TREATMENT

- In an unco-operative patient give 1 mg of glucagon i.m. which works in 10–15 min.
- If treatment is delayed for any reason, recovery may be slow due to the development of cerebral oedema; dexamethasone 12 mg stat i.v. has been suggested in these patients.
- Once the patient is conscious give him something to eat. Watch for relapse particularly in patients taking the long-acting sulphonylurea preparations.

DIABETIC KETOACIDOSIS

Signs
Impaired consciousness, dehydration, hyperventilation, and smell of acetone

Investigations
Immediately
    – blood glucose, U+E.
    – pH, pCO_2, pO_2.
later
    – FBC
    – ECG, chest X-ray
    – blood, urine and throat swab for culture.

TREATMENT

1. Fluids
    Commence i.v. infusion of N saline.
        1 litre in 30 min
        1 litre in 1 hour
        1 litre in 2 hours
        1 litre in 4 hours
    If the sodium level rises >150 mmol/l change to 1/2 normal saline.

2. Insulin
    Give 10 units of soluble or Actrapid insulin by i.v. injection (Actrapid if the patient is a new diabetic or is already on monocomponent insulins) Give an intravenous infusion of a short acting insulin 6 units per hour. If a continuous infusion pump is not available use hourly i.m. injections of 6 units of insulin. If the blood sugar fails to fall increase the dose to 12 units hourly.

3. Potassium
    Start to replace potassium losses early before the level starts to fall. Give 20 mmol/hour of potassium in the i.v. fluids as soon as the first dose of insulin has been given. Increase to 40 mmol/hr if the serum potassium is low (<4 mmol/l). If the potassium rises above 6 mmol/l stop the potassium addition. ECG monitoring allows warning of extreme changes in potassium levels.

4. Bicarbonate
    If the patient's pH <7.0 give 100 mmol of sodium bicarbonate
    (DO NOT use the 8.4% solution) over 20 min.
    Repeat blood gases.
    Repeat dose of bicarbonate if pH still <7.0
    Monitor the potassium level when giving bicarbonate as it may
    fall rapidly.

5. Nasogastric tube
    All patients who are unconscious or semi-conscious should have
    a nasogastric tube passed and the stomach contents emptied.
    Gastric atony is frequent and carries a risk of aspiration.

6. Hypotension
    If the patient is persistently hypotensive (systolic <80 mmHg for
    2 hours) give 2 units of plasma or whole blood, then review.

7. Precipitating factors
    Look for factors which may have precipitated ketoacidosis, such
    as infection (especially throat, urine and chest) and myocardial
    infarction. Abdominal tenderness may be due to diabetic
    ketoacidosis, or an acute abdomen may precipitate ketoacidosis.
    Therefore, any patient with abdominal tenderness must be
    monitored very carefully for other signs of an acute abdomen,
    such as guarding.

8. Urinary catheter
    Pass a urinary catheter only if no urine is produced after 4 hours
    of treatment.

9. CVP
    Consider the use of a CVP line in patients with cardiac disease.

10. Subsequent management
    When the blood glucose falls to below 15 mmol/l change to 5%
    dextrose 1 l every 6 hours and reduce the rate of insulin infusion
    to 3 units/hour. Further reduction depends on an individual
    patient's requirements. Continue the 5% dextrose infusion and
    insulin infusion until the patient is eating his normal diet.
    The rapid determination of blood glucose by Dextrostix and
    Ames meter or by B.M. 20–800 strip have made sliding scales of
    insulin obsolete in the transition from continuous infusion of
    insulin to intermittent injections.
    Change to 4 hourly s.c. injections of one of the short-acting

insulins. The initial dose depends on the previous requirements but is usually in the range of 12–20 units; subsequent doses depend on the blood glucose level measured shortly before the dose is due and the response to the previous dose.

Gradually amalgamate the doses of insulin until the patient is back on a b.d. regime which should be in a similar range to that prior to admission, but take into account the insulin requirements of the previous 24 hours. Note that frequent small doses of insulin are more effective than the same total dose given as large infrequent injections.

11. Failure of clinical improvement

If the clinical improvement is not as fast as expected consider co-existing conditions such as: cerebrovascular accident, Addison's disease, meningitis, myocardial infarction, hypo-glycaemia (over-treatment).

HYPEROSMOLAR HYPERGLYCAEMIC NON-KETOTIC COMA

This occurs in elderly non-insulin dependent diabetics in whom it may be the first presentation of diabetes.

The management of hyperosmolar coma is similar to ketoacidosis but with certain provisos:

1. the insulin requirements are often small.

2. the serum sodium level is frequently >150 mmol/l at presentation and requires the use of 1/2 normal saline.

3. anticoagulate the patient with heparin as the risk of thrombosis is high.

4. a CVP line is frequently indicated in view of the age of the majority of these patients.

LACTIC ACIDOSIS

This is a rare cause of acidosis in the diabetic and should be suspected in:

- a diabetic who is acidotic but who has little or no ketonuria.
- any diabetic on treatment with a biguanide particularly phenformin.
- an acidotic patient with a large anion gap. If the sodium concentration minus the chloride and bicarbonate concentrations is >15 mmol it suggests that a significant amount of another anion is circulating, i.e. lactate.

If there is any suspicion that lactic acidosis may be present its presence should be confirmed by measuring blood lactate level.

Management

1. Correct the dehydration, hyperglycaemia and hypovolaemia as for diabetic ketoacidosis.

2. Attempt to correct the acidosis by the use of large quantities of bicarbonate. Give 200 mmol of bicarbonate (in dilute solution eg. 1.26%) over 30 min then repeat test for pH and bicarbonate level. Continue infusing bicarbonate until the pH and bicarbonate level start to return towards normal.

Diabetes and Surgery

PATIENTS ON ORAL HYPOGLYCAEMIC DRUGS

1. Stop the oral hypoglycaemic agent on the day of surgery.

2. Check the blood glucose prior to theatre and commence i.v. infusion of 5% dextrose if the glucose level is low (only likely to occur if the patient is on a long-acting agent such as chlorpropamide).

3. Post-operatively monitor the blood sugar frequently using standard lab tests or, more conveniently, Dextrostix and meter or B.M. 20–800 sticks. Some patients may require insulin for a short period post-operatively. If so, start with small doses of a short-acting insulin (8–12 units) and adjust the dose according to the response.

4. Restart on an oral hypoglycaemic agent as soon as the patient is eating.

INSULIN DEPENDENT DIABETICS

1. Arrange for surgery to take place as early as possible during the day.

2. Arrange for the patient to be admitted for stabilisation (48 hours) on a b.d. dosage of a short-acting insulin prior to surgery.

3. On the day of surgery commence an infusion of 5% dextrose (1 l over 4 hours) at 8.00 am.

4. Give half the normal morning dosage of a short-acting insulin.

5. Check the blood sugar before theatre and if <6.0 mmol/l give 20 ml of 50% dextrose i.v.

6. The blood glucose should be checked during surgery if the operation is major and immediately post-operatively in any case and every 2–3 hours until stable.

7. Continue the 5% dextrose infusion until the patient is eating normally.

8. Use frequent (4 hourly) injections of a short-acting insulin over the immediate post-operative period.

9. As an alternative to the above regime, a continuous infusion of insulin at 2–3 units/hour together with 5% dextrose 1 l in 4 hours may be used. If staff are unfamiliar with continuous infusion pumps, or there are problems with drips running to time, a regime in which the insulin is included in the dextrose can be used.
    – commence infusion of 10% dexrose containing 15 units of Actrapid insulin per 500 ml bag at a rate of 100 ml/hour.
    – check blood glucose every 2–3 hours.
    – if the blood glucose < 5 mmol/l change to 5 units of Actrapid per bag.
    – if > 10 mmol/l change to 20 units per bag.

10. Once the patient is eating normally, change back to normal dose of insulin, this may need to be increased as he is likely to be less active in hospital.

10. Good control is important over the post-operative period for any type of diabetic as the wound healing is better if control is good.

SUGGESTED READING

1. *Medicine Series* 4 1981 No. 6–9
    Medical Education (International)

2. R. Hall, J. Anderson, G.A. Smart, M. Besser.
    Fundamentals of Clinical Endocrinology 3rd Ed. 1981

9

HAEMATOLOGY

Diagnosis of Anaemia

Anaemia is defined as a haemoglobin < 13 g/dl in men and < 11.5 g/dl in women.

Full blood count, blood film and reticulocyte count are essential investigations in all cases of anaemia.

Polycythaemia

DEFINITION

– Hb > 18.0 g/dl or PCV > 0.55 or RBC > 5.5 x 10^9/l in men
– Hb > 17.0 g/dl or PCV > 0.52 or RBC > 5.0 x 10^9/l in women

CAUSES

1. Relative polycythaemia, where the increase in PCV is caused by a reduction in plasma volume. Red cell mass is normal.
    (a) dehydration. Assess clinically and from history, fluid balance, etc.
    (b) "stress" polycythaemia. Almost 50% fall into this group.
         A typical patient is obese, hypertensive and a smoker, with vascular disease. The mechanism is unclear.

2. True polycythaemia, where the red cell mass is raised (>35 ml/kg in males, >32 ml/kg in females) but other features of primary polycythaemia (see below) are absent.
    (a) chronic hypoxia – in chest disease, cyanotic heart disease, high altitude, hypoventilation.
         Investigations – arterial blood gases, chest X-ray, pulmonary function tests.

NORMOCYTIC ANAEMIA

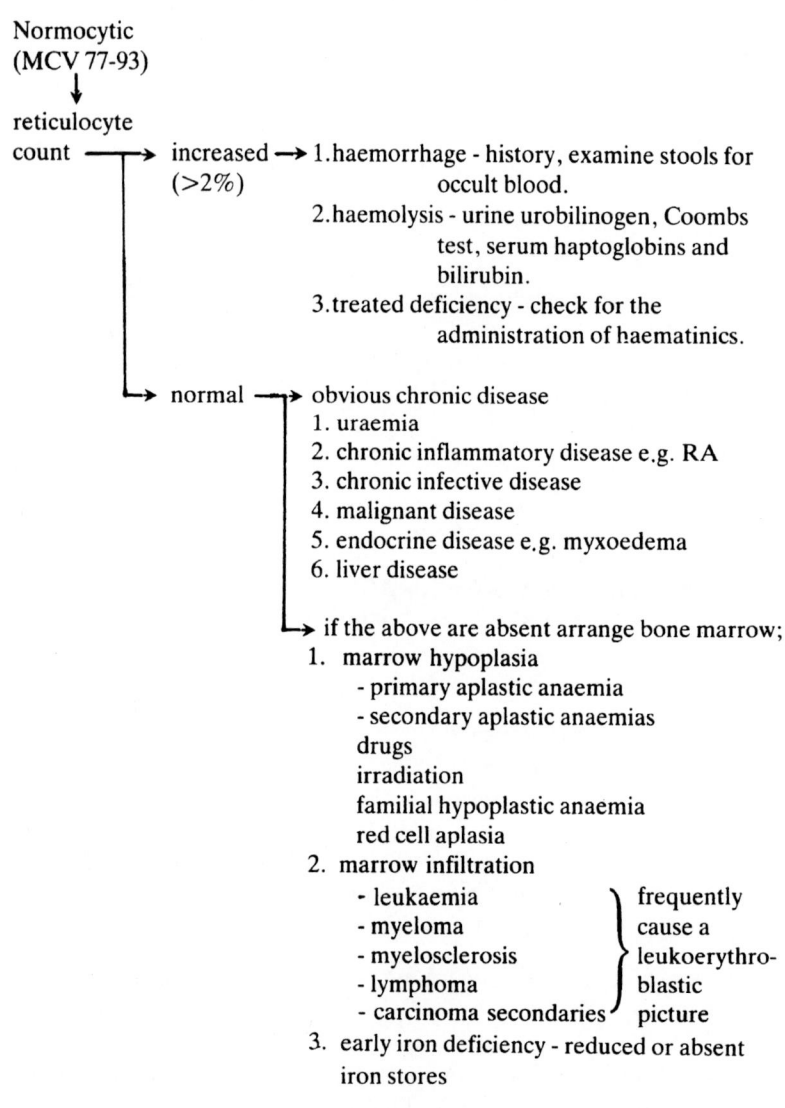

Normocytic
(MCV 77-93)
↓
reticulocyte
count ────→ increased ──→ 1. haemorrhage - history, examine stools for
              (>2%)   occult blood.
                           2. haemolysis - urine urobilinogen, Coombs
                                       test, serum haptoglobins and
                                       bilirubin.
                           3. treated deficiency - check for the
                                       administration of haematinics.

        ↳ normal ──→ obvious chronic disease
                     1. uraemia
                     2. chronic inflammatory disease e.g. RA
                     3. chronic infective disease
                     4. malignant disease
                     5. endocrine disease e.g. myxoedema
                     6. liver disease

                   ↳ if the above are absent arrange bone marrow;
                     1. marrow hypoplasia
                          - primary aplastic anaemia
                          - secondary aplastic anaemias
                          drugs
                          irradiation
                          familial hypoplastic anaemia
                          red cell aplasia
                     2. marrow infiltration
                          - leukaemia   } frequently
                          - myeloma   cause a
                          - myelosclerosis   leukoerythro-
                          - lymphoma   blastic
                          - carcinoma secondaries   picture
                     3. early iron deficiency - reduced or absent
                          iron stores

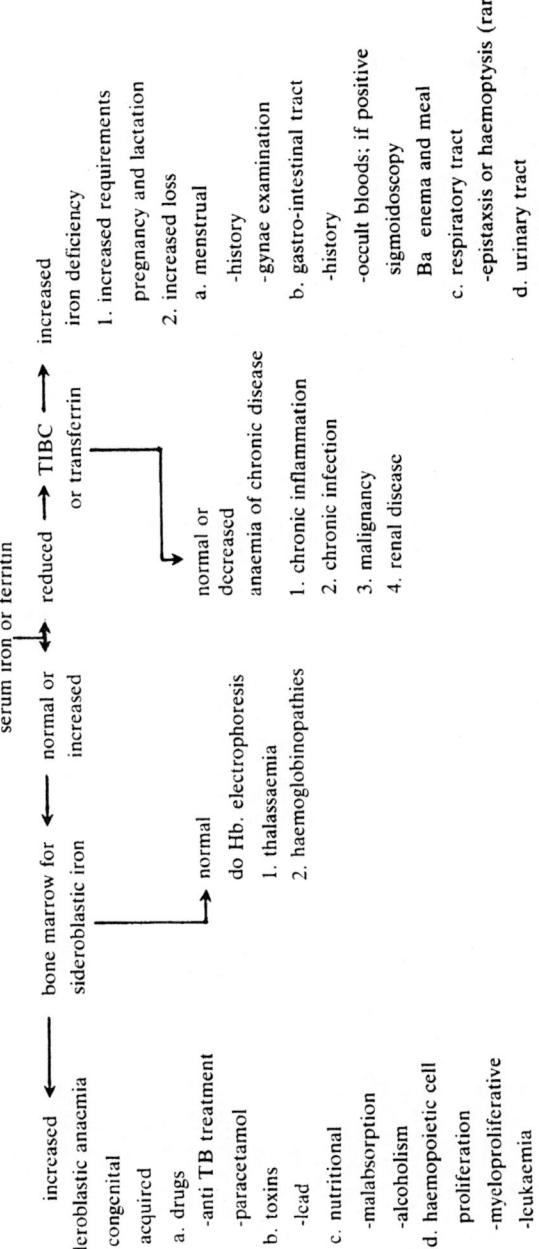

MICROCYTIC ANAEMIA

Microcytic (MCV<77)

serum iron or ferritin

increased → bone marrow for sideroblastic iron

normal

increased
sideroblastic anaemia
1. congenital
2. acquired
 a. drugs
  -anti TB treatment
  -paracetamol
 b. toxins
  -lcad
 c. nutritional
  -malabsorption
  -alcoholism
 d. haemopoietic cell proliferation
  -myeloproliferative
  -leukaemia

normal or increased

do Hb. electrophoresis
1. thalassaemia
2. haemoglobinopathies

reduced → TIBC or transferrin

normal or decreased
anaemia of chronic disease
1. chronic inflammation
2. chronic infection
3. malignancy
4. renal disease

increased

iron deficiency
1. increased requirements
 pregnancy and lactation
2. increased loss
 a. menstrual
  -history
  -gynae examination
 b. gastro-intestinal tract
  -history
  -occult bloods; if positive
   sigmoidoscopy
   Ba enema and meal
 c. respiratory tract
  -epistaxsis or haemoptysis (rare)
 d. urinary tract
 e. coagulation defects
3. impaired absorption
 gastric surgery, coeliac disease

MACROCYTIC ANAEMIA

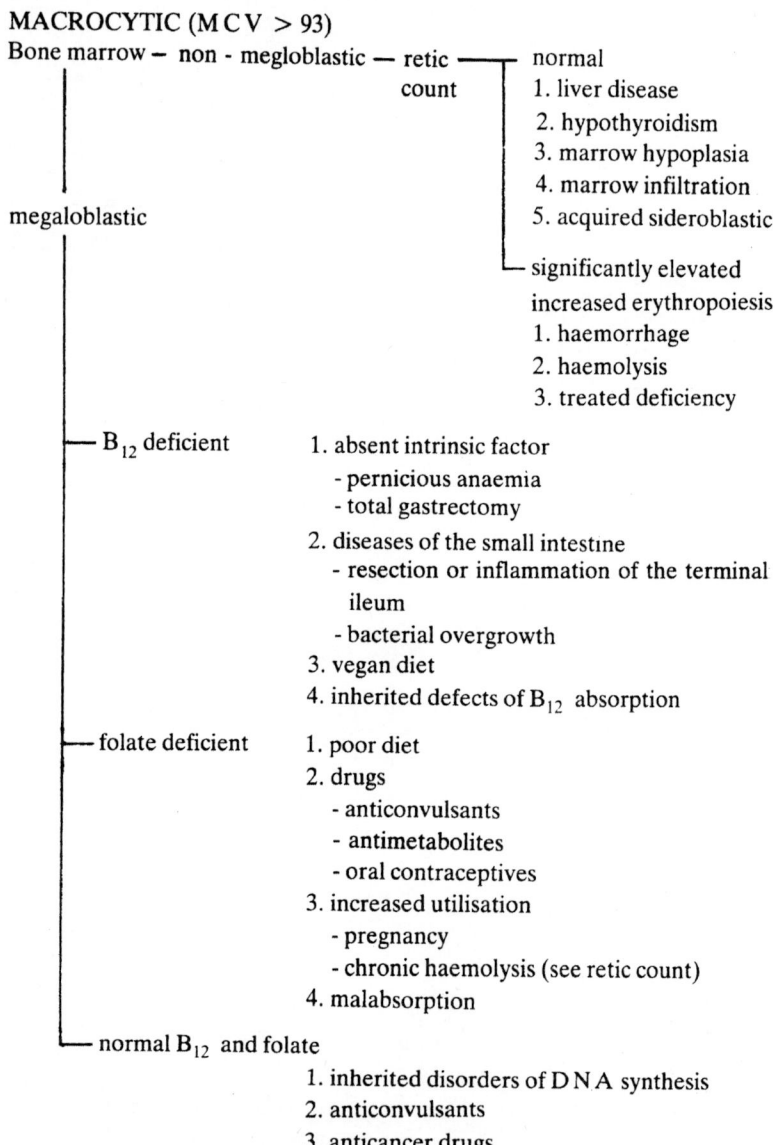

MACROCYTIC (M C V > 93)

Bone marrow — non - megloblastic — retic count —

normal
1. liver disease
2. hypothyroidism
3. marrow hypoplasia
4. marrow infiltration
5. acquired sideroblastic

significantly elevated increased erythropoiesis
1. haemorrhage
2. haemolysis
3. treated deficiency

megaloblastic

— B_{12} deficient
1. absent intrinsic factor
   - pernicious anaemia
   - total gastrectomy
2. diseases of the small intestine
   - resection or inflammation of the terminal ileum
   - bacterial overgrowth
3. vegan diet
4. inherited defects of B_{12} absorption

— folate deficient
1. poor diet
2. drugs
   - anticonvulsants
   - antimetabolites
   - oral contraceptives
3. increased utilisation
   - pregnancy
   - chronic haemolysis (see retic count)
4. malabsorption

— normal B_{12} and folate
1. inherited disorders of D N A synthesis
2. anticonvulsants
3. anticancer drugs

Treatment – the benefits of venesection are less marked in this group but, if the patient is symptomatic, improvement may be expected if the PCV is reduced below 0.50.

(b) inappropriate erythropoetin production

- renal carcinoma
- hydrorephrosis   } arrange IVP
- renal cysts   and test urine.

- hepatoma : liver scan, biopsy, alpha-fetoprotein
- cerebellar haemangioblastoma : examine for cerebellar signs and evidence of raised intra-cranial pressure
- other causes include: uterine fibroids, phaeochromocytoma.

Treatment – once the cause is established, and if surgery is contemplated, it is better to reduce the haematocrit by venesection before operation.

(c) Primary – Polycythaemia Rubra Vera (primary proliferative polycythaemia) usually presents with thrombotic (arterial or venous) or haemorrhagic complications. The patients are often hypertensive and may have associated gout or peptic ulceration. Splenomegaly is common. If the patient has developed haemorrhagic complications, particularly GIT bleeding, he may have a hypochromic, microcytic anaemia. WBC and platelet count are frequently raised, as are serum urate and neutrophil alkaline phosphatase (NAP).

Treatment
- venesection, remove 500 ml at a time (more if replaced with i.v. dextran).
- can be repeated after 24 hours if rapid reduction of haematocrit is required.
- aim to reduce the PCV to 0.45.
- with ischaemic symptoms or raised platelet count replace with dextran infusion.

White Blood Cell Counts

LEUKOCYTOSIS

1. infection.

2. haemorrhage, uraemia, diabetic acidosis, myocardial infarction,

steroids, malignancy, trauma, surgery, following an epileptic fit
or paroxysmal tachycardia.

3.   myeloproliferative disease

LEUKAEMOID REACTION

Neutrophil count > 30,000

1.   disseminated malignancy (especially liver and marrow).

2.   severe infection (especially following splenectomy).

3.   miliary tuberculosis.

The main differential diagnosis is chronic myeloid leukaemia. In a
leukaemoid reaction there are mature neutrophils but no blast cells in
the peripheral blood, a high leukocyte alkaline phosphatase (low in
CML), no Philadelphia chromosome and splenomegaly is rare.

NEUTROPENIA

Acute
      – virus infections
      – bacteria: TB, brucella, typhoid, septicaemia
      – following blood transfusion.
Prolonged
      – aplastic anaemia, acute leukaemia, and marrow infiltration
      – hypersplenism
      – SLE
      – drugs: phenylbutazone, indomethacin, co-trimoxazole, dap-
        sone, carbimazole, chlorpromazine, chloramphenicol,
        cytotoxics, gold, penicillamine.

LYMPHOCYTOSIS

Viral infections, TB, brucellosis, chronic lymphatic leukaemia.

MONOCYTOSIS

Glandular fever, brucellosis, malaria, toxoplasmosis, SBE, TB,
malignant disease.

EOSINOPHILIA

      – parasitic infections
      – asthma, pulmonary eosinophilia (in association with pulmonary

infiltrates on chest X-ray)
- drug reactions
- Hodgkin's disease and carcinomatosis
- polyarteritis nodosa.

Virus infections, myxoedema, allergy, CML, PRV.

Erythrocyte Sedimentation Rate

Raised in
- infection
- inflammation
- connective tissue diseases
- malignancy
- anaemia
- chronic renal disease
- bleeding
- pregnancy

If no obvious cause found consider:
- UTI
- myeloma
- SBE
- giant cell arteritis

Very low in
- polycythaemia
- congestive cardiac failure
- liver failure

Disseminated Intravascular Coagulation

CAUSES

- severe bacterial (meningococcal, staphylococcal, and gram negative) and viral infections.
- obstetric problems: antepartum haemorrhage, amniotic fluid embolism.
- malignancy: adenocarcinoma, prostatic carcinoma, acute promyelocytic leukaemia.
- trauma or surgery.
- others: liver failure, anaphylaxis, incompatible blood transfusion

EFFECTS

– haemorrhage especially into skin, venepuncture sites and GIT.
– renal failure, jaundice, cardio-respiratory failure.

INVESTIGATIONS

Early –blood film shows fragmented red cells , fibrin degradation
      products are increased, thrombin clotting time is prolonged.
Later –other abnormalities on the clotting screen, thrombocytopenia.
Severe –low fibrinogen, prolonged prothrombin time and accelerated
      partial thromboplastin time.

MANAGEMENT

1. Treat underlying disease.
2. Heparin – see "PE/DVT".
3. Fresh frozen plasma and platelet concentrates (but only if heparin
    has been given).

Haemolysis

INVESTIGATIONS

FBC – anaemia, reticulocytosis.
Blood film – many abnormal RBC types which may be diagnostic or
      give a clue to the cause.
Biochemistry – unconjugated bilirubin (increased), LDH (increased),
      haptoglobins (reduced or absent), plasma protein elec-
      trophoresis.
Urine – increased urobilinogen.
Coombs test.
Warm or cold antibodies.
Mycoplasma complement fixation test.
Intravascular haemolysis produces – haemoglobinuria, haemo-
      globinaemia, urinary haemosiderin and fragmented red
      cells.

CAUSES

1. Inherited abnormalities of
    (a) haemoglobin
            – thalassaemia, sickle cell disease

Hb electrophoresis
(b) enzymes
- G6PD deficiency (precipitated by drugs).
enzyme assay.
(c) membranes
- hereditary spherocytosis, eliptocytosis
blood film, osmotic fragility.

2. Intravascular
(a) heart valve prosthesis.
(b) microangiopathic haemolytic anaemia
- septicaemia, DIC.
(c) falciparum malaria
- Blackwater fever.
(d) paroxysmal nocturnal haemoglobinuria (gives positive Ham's test).

3. Autoimmune (Coombs positive)
- primary
- secondary
(a) warm antibody: lymphomas, CLL, SLE
(b) cold antibody: viral infections, mycoplasma
(c) drugs: methyl dopa, high dose penicillin, hydralazine, cephalothin etc.

Bleeding Disorders

1. Vascular defects
- purpura is common but serious haemorrhage is rare.
Causes
- old age, steroids, septicaemia, and other infections, scurvy, uraemia, Henoch-Schonlein purpura.
Investigations
- platelet count, PT (prothrombin time), and APPT (accelerated partial thromboplastin time) all normal. Bleeding time may be prolonged.

2. Platelet defects
- bruising rare unless count $< 50 \times 10^9/1$
Causes
(a) primary (idiopathic thrombocytopaenic purpura).
(b) secondary- aplastic anaemia, leukaemia, cytotoxic drugs, myeloma, marrow replacement.

       – drugs (immune or marrow depression).
       – SLE, infection (usually viral).
       – DIC, massive transfusion.
       – splenomegaly.

Investigation
     – platelet count reduced, bleeding time prolonged. PT and
      APPT normal.

Treatment
     – remove cause.
     – in emergency consider platelet transfusion (benefit is very
      transient if there is an immune mechanism).
     – in ITP consider high dose steroids and, if chronic, consider
      splenectomy.

3.   Coagulation defects
     Causes
    (a) inherited: haemophilia, Christmas disease
    (b) acquired: warfarin, heparin, liver disease, malabsorption,
        DIC.
     Investigation
       – bleeding time and platelet count normal.
       – APTT prolonged.
       – PT often prolonged (not in haemophilia).
       – specific assay of clotting factors may be indicated.
     For investigation of DIC see "Disseminated Intravascular
     Coagulation"

POST OPERATIVE BLEEDING

1.   Exclude a surgical cause of bleeding.

2.   Transfuse to correct shock, hypotension, or anaemia.

3.   Exclude anticoagulant effect of drugs.

4.   Give vitamin K_1 i.v. if there is a possibility of a deficiency.

5.   Give fresh frozen plasma if a large transfusion is being given.

6.   Check platelet count and if reduced, consider possible causes.

7.   Consider the possibility of DIC and investigate as necessary.

8.   Post prostatectomy, aminocaproic acid is often useful.

Causes of Splenomegaly

COMMON

Minor – infectious mononucleosis, infective endocarditis, collagen diseases.
Moderate – acute leukaemia, portal hypertension, malaria, CLL, lymphoma.
Massive – CML, myelofibrosis, kala-azar.

LESS COMMON

Haematological – ITP, PRV, haemolytic anaemia, pernicious anaemia, iron deficiency.
Infective – typhoid, septicaemia, brucellosis, viral hepatitis.
Miscellaneous –
        SLE, secondary amyloidosis, sarcoidosis, thyrotoxicosis, rheumatoid arthritis (Felty's syndrome), lipoidosis.

SUGGESTED READING

1.   *Medicine Series 3* 1980 No. 27–29
      Medical Education (International)

2.   R.B. Thompson
      A Short Textbook of Haematology 5th Ed. 1979
      Pitman Medical

10

RHEUMATOLOGY

Rheumatoid Arthritis

CLINICAL FEATURES

A sub-acute or chronic inflammatory destructive polyarthritis, with peripheral, symmetrical joint involvement. In the acute stages the joints are tender and warm with synovial proliferation and effusions. Rheumatoid nodules and kerato-conjunctivitis sicca occur in some cases.

DIFFERENTIAL DIAGNOSIS

- osteoarthritis; typically involving the terminal interphalangeal joints (TIP), the carpo-metacarpal joint of the thumb and the large weight-bearing joints of the lower limb.
- psoriatic arthritis; this occurs in several forms, the most common involving the TIP joints. Another form involves the metacarpophalangeal and proximal interphalangeal joints but is less symmetrical than rheumatoid arthritis.
- reactive arthritis; this term is given to a number of post-infective forms of arthritis, but it is typically a relatively short-lived, non-destructive polyarthritis.
- systemic lupus erythematosus; amongst the most common of its many features there is a non-deforming non-destructive polyarthritis.
- gout; may present as a polyarthritis rather than the more familiar acutely inflamed, extremely painful monoarthritis although there is usually a history of more typical episodes.

MANAGEMENT OF RHEUMATOID ARTHRITIS

Patient Education

Rheumatoid arthritis is a long term disease and the patient's attitude to the disease is frequently as important as any drug treatment. The general public's ideas about rheumatoid arthritis are often unduly pessimistic, and should be corrected.

It is important to prevent flexion deformities, particularly of the knee. These arise because the position of comfort for a patient with a painful knee is with the knee bent and the back of the knee supported. This may be comfortable but rapidly leads to the knee being fixed in a flexed position, which is very poor functionally.

Drug Treatment

The "first line" treatment of rheumatoid arthritis is one of the non-steroidal anti-inflammatory drugs, which are similar to aspirin in their actions. There are now over 30 available, from which a selection of 3 or 4 will cover the majority of requirements. They should be used singly, in the minimum dose to produce relief of symptoms.If no improvement is produced when the drug is first introduced it should be increased to the maximum dose allowed, before being replaced with another. There is considerable variability between patients and their reponse to this group of drugs. It is, therefore, reasonable to try several of these drugs in sequence then allow the patient to decide which he finds the most effective. A 7–10 day period is normally long enough to judge whether a drug is effective.

Some of the commonly used first line drugs include:
 – indomethacin 25–50 mg t.d.s. or q.d.s.
 – naproxen 250–500 mg t.d.s.
 – ibuprofen 400–600 mg t.d.s. or q.d.s.
 – piroxicam 20 mg daily.

The princjpal "second line" drugs in rheumatoid arthritis are gold and penicillamine. They alter the basic disease process, whereas the first line drugs are purely symptomatic treatment. The majority of patients with rheumatoid arthritis can be controlled on first line drugs. Second line drugs are indicated when progressive rheumatoid arthritis is not controlled by first line drugs.

In contrast to the first line drugs which are relatively safe, the second line drugs have potentially lethal side-effects, and therefore require careful monitoring. They also differ markedly from the first line drugs in their time course of action which is over months rather than hours.

Assessment prior to treatment with gold or penicillamine:
- FBC, ESR, differential WBC and platelets.
- U+E's.
- urine for blood and protein

Side-effects of gold and penicillamine are skin rashes, stomatitis, thrombocytopaenia, agranulocytosis, aplastic anaemia, proteinuria and haematuria.

Schedule for treatment with gold:
- give a 10 mg test dose of myocrisin i.m.
- check urine (for blood and protein), platelets and white cell count
- then if no reaction give 50 mg i.m. weekly.
- reduce to fortnightly then monthly injections once a response to treatment has occurred. Review the therapy when 1 g of gold in total has been given. If there has been no demonstrable improvement on clinical grounds or laboratory parameters (ESR etc.) discontinue the gold.
- if a response has been produced continue the gold on a maintenance basis in a dose of 50 mg monthly.
- stop treatment if any of the above side-effects develop.

Treatment with penicillamine:
- if assessment clear (see above).
- commence on a dose of 250 mg daily.
- check FBC, platelets, differential white count and urine every 2 weeks.
- increase the dose by 250 mg every 2 months to a maximum of 750 mg daily if side-effects allow, continuing at the minimum dose at which a response is achieved.
- if no response is achieved after 2 months on 750 mg daily stop the treatment.
- if side-effects develop stop treatment.

Acute Monoarthritis

A patient with an acutely painful, swollen, red joint must be considered to have a septic arthritis until proven otherwise, and the joint aspirated immediately. The differential diagnosis includes the crystal diseases (gout and calcium pyrophosphate arthropathy) and haemarthrosis.

SEPTIC ARTHRITIS

Synovial fluid obtained should be sent for:
- – immediate Gram stain.
- – culture and sensitivity (including AFBs).
- – microscopy (including polarising light microscopy for crystals).
- – X-rays of the affected joint (as a baseline).

Also send blood cultures and look carefully for any other sites of infection, such as skin and urinary tract.

Beware of the patient with rheumatoid arthritis who develops a single painful joint; this should be aspirated as these patients are particularly liable to develop septic arthritis.

Management
1. Aspirate the joint to make the diagnosis.

2. Splint the affected joint in a position of function (eg. straight for the knee and flexed for the elbow).

3. Cefuroxime 1 g t.d.s. i.m., continue until the culture results are available when change to more specific antibiotics, and continue antibiotic treatment for a total of 6 weeks.

4. Give adequate analgesia.

5. If no culture results are available change after 7 days to broad spectrum oral antibiotics such as ampicillin and flucloxacillin to complete the course.

6. Repeat aspiration if the joint remains swollen.

GOUT

Gout usually presents as an acute, very painful, small joint monoarthritis, 70% of attacks involving the great toe.

Causes
1. Primary
   - – hereditary, family history.

2. Secondary
   - – drugs: diuretics (thiazide and loop), low dose aspirin.
   - – tissue destruction eg. following cytotoxic drug treatment.

Treatment
1. Confirm the diagnosis by aspiration of the affected joint.

2. Commence indomethacin 50 mg q.d.s. or naproxen 500 mg t.d.s. Continue treatment for several days after the symptoms have settled.

3. Consider using prophylactic treatment in patients with recurrent acute episodes or in patients who are getting chronic attacks of gout.
    Allopurinol 300 mg daily, increasing to a maximum of 600 mg daily if lower doses fail to prevent further episodes, is an extremely effective prophylactic treatment.
    Do not start allopurinol within 6 weeks of an acute attack. It is wise when commencing allopurinol to give indomethacin or naproxen as well for a few weeks to reduce the likelihood of an acute attack.

Paget's Disease

CLINICAL FEATURES

Include bone pain (continuous aching), nocturnal pain, tenderness and warmth over involved areas, deformity (bowing of tibia, flattening of the skull), pathological fractures, cranial nerve entrapment, and osteosarcoma in <1% of cases.

INVESTIGATIONS

- alkaline phosphatase (considerably elevated).
- calcium (elevated only if the patient is immobilised).
- X-rays: osteosclerosis, osteoporosis, widened cortices, loss of trabecular pattern.
- 24 hour urinary hydroxyproline excretion (elevated due to increased bone turnover).

INDICATIONS FOR TREATMENT

- bone pain
- neurological complications
- delayed fracture healing
- immobilisation hypercalcaemia
- before and after orthopaedic surgery on involved areas.

TREATMENT

1. Calcitonin 0.5–2.0 units/kg daily i.m.. Once improvement is noted reduce frequency of injections to three times weekly and continue for 3–6 months then withdraw and observe.
   Calcitonin administered in a prolonged course is immunogenic. Salcatonin 50 units three times weekly can be substituted if problems arise.

2. Diphosphonates are stable analogues of pyrophosphate which coat the surface of mineral bone preventing normal osteoclast activity. Disodium etridonate is the most commonly used diphosphonate in a dose of 5 mg/kg/day for a course of 3–6 months. In high dosage it may produce osteomalacia.

3. Mithramycin is a cytotoxic antibiotic which is thought to have a direct effect on osteoclasts. In doses of 25 μg/kg weekly or less frequently it is effective in reducing bone pain but has potential hepatic, renal and haematological side-effects which limit its use.

SUGGESTED READING

1. *Medicine 4th series* No. 10–11 1981
   Medical Education (International)

2. J.T. Scott
   Copeman's Textbook of the Rheumatic Diseases 5th Ed. 1978
   Churchill Livingstone

11

DRUG OVERDOSE

Management

The basic principles of management of a patient with self poisoning are the same as for any patient whose level of consciousness is reduced.

- maintain airway and ventilation.
- general care of the unconscious patient. Nurse in "coma" position.
- assess and record degree of coma.
- check cardiovascular status (BP, peripheral perfusion, arrhythymias).
- check temperature (patients with drug overdoses may have hypothermia).
- assess hydration.

In addition it is of value to obtain as much information as possible from relatives, friends, ambulance men etc. about what drugs may have been taken. This serves as a useful rough guide, but too much importance should not be placed on it as the information is frequently unreliable.

GASTRIC LAVAGE

If the patient is admitted within 4 hours of ingestion of drugs, gastric lavage should be considered. The time limit is extended to 8 hours in the case of aspirin or antidepressants with an atropine-like effect. Gastric lavage should not be considered a routine procedure as its effectiveness is debatable and it does carry some risks, particularly when performed by inexperienced staff.

Gastric lavage should not be used in the following circumstances:

- an unco-operative patient.
- a patient with poor or absent cough reflex, unless an

endotracheal tube is passed first.

– where corrosives or caustics have been ingested (risk of perforation).

– where paraffin or petrol have been ingested (risk of aspiration).

Complications of gastric lavage: aspiration, mis-directed tube, oral, dental and oesophageal damage.

When the procedure is carried out it should be done by staff experienced in the procedure, with a co-operative patient, with an intact gag reflex or ET tube. Lie the patient on her side, tilted head down, and use a well lubricated wide bore tube.

EMESIS

Ipecacuanha syrup is frequently used in children, and its use in adults in a dose of 30 ml, repeated after 20 min if there is no result, can also be effective. Other emetics are unreliable and potentially unsafe and should not be used.

SPECIFIC ANTIDOTES

Few drugs have specific antidotes, some of the more common ones include:

opiates – naloxone
paracetamol – cysteamine, N-acetylcysteine or methionine
iron salts – desferrioxamine.

PSYCHIATRIC FEATURES

Few patients who are admitted to hospital following an overdose of drugs have a formal psychiatric illness. However, an interview with a psychiatrist should be arranged for all patients before they are discharged, as there is evidence that this reduces the rate of recurrence, and improves the chances of detecting those with true psychiatric illness.

NATIONAL POISONS INFORMATION SERVICE

The National Poisons Information centres provide useful information about the effects and treatment of poisonings. They are particularly useful when unusual substances are taken accidentally or deliberately.

London 01 407 7600
Belfast 0232 30503
Cardiff 0222 492233
Dublin 0001 745588

Edinburgh 031 229 2477
Leeds 0532 32799
Manchester 061 740 2254
Newcastle 0632 325131

Treatment of Salicylate Poisoning

Typical features include: restlessness and confusion, sweating, hyperventilation, tinnitus, coma (rarely in salicylate poisoning alone). A variety of biochemical features may be present due to vomiting, hyperventilation and the acidity of the drug.

INVESTIGATIONS

- blood gases
- U+E
- Measure salicylate level

>1.9 mmol/l (30mg%) symptomatic poisoning

>3.1 mmol/l severe poisoning

>6.2 mmol/l indication for treatment with haemoperfusion or haemodialysis if available.

Forced alkaline diuresis is indicated in patients with symptomatic poisoning or worse, who have normal or relatively normal renal function.

Forced alkaline diuresis regime

1.26% sodium bicarbonate		
	1/2 litre	Give over 2 hours
5% dextrose	1/2 litre	Check the urine pH which
N.saline	1/2 litre	should become alkaline,
5% dextrose	1/2 litre	if not double bicarbonate.

Potassium supplements should be incorporated into the regime initially at 20 mmol/hour then depending on the serum potassium which should be monitored 4 hourly during the diuresis.

Paracetamol Poisoning

Self poisoning with paracetamol, either taken alone or in combination with other drugs such as opiate derivatives, is common and potentially lethal. As few as 16 tablets (8 g) have proved fatal. The danger is not in the early stages which are relatively mild, but in the late development of liver damage and renal failure (primary or secondary to liver failure).

Specific treatment needs to be given within 10 hours of ingestion of the drug. The decision whether specific treatment is required depends on the plasma paracetamol level at 4 hours or longer following ingestion.

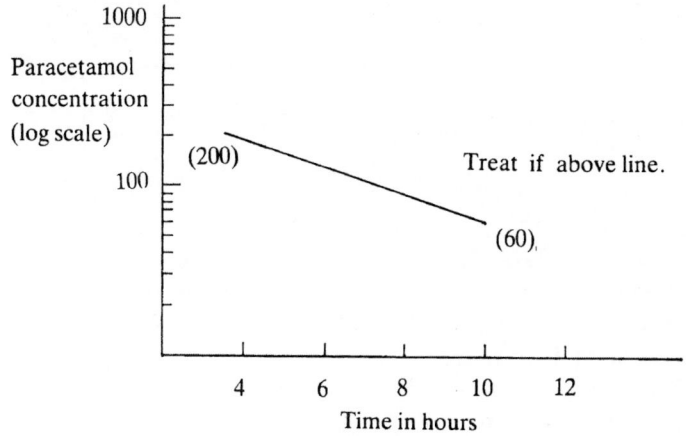

1. Cysteamine 2 g i.v. over 10 min
   Then 800 mg as an i.v. infusion over 4 hours
   800 mg as an i.v. infusion over 16 hours
   Cysteamine is being replaced in some centres by N-acetylcysteine because of the frequent side-effects such as nausea and vomiting, and the difficulties involved in its storage and sterility.

OR

2. N-acetylcysteine, initially 150 mg/kg over 15 min as an i.v. injection, followed by 50 mg/kg in 500 ml of 5% dextrose over 4 hours and 100 mg/kg in 1 litre of 5% dextrose over 16 hours. The much reduced toxicity of n-acetylcysteine compared with cysteamine allows its use on suspicion of a significant overdose before the paracetamol level is available to confirm this.

OR

3. Methionine is effective and less toxic than cysteamine, but its oral administration in patients who are nauseated and vomiting does not guarantee effective absorption.
   Methionine 2.5 g stat.
   Followed by 2.5 g at 4 hourly intervals for 3 doses.

Benzodiazepines

These drugs are frequently taken in overdosage but rarely cause significant problems, unless the patient also has respiratory disease when respiratory depression can occur.

Barbiturates

These drugs are now less readily available, but overdoses still occur either deliberately or as part of drug abuse.
Evidence for severe poisoning
- deep coma
- hypotension
- poor respiratory effort
- a rapidly deteriorating level of consciousness
- blood barbiturate levels >0.21 mmol/l (5 mg/100 ml) for short or medium acting drugs and >0.43 mmol/l (10 mg/100 ml) for phenobarbitone.

Treatment
- general supportive measures
- forced diuresis.

severe cases
- forced alkaline diuresis for phenobarbitone (see salicylate poisoning)
- charcoal haemoperfusion if available is indicated in severely poisoned patients.

Iron

Iron is often taken as an accidental overdose by children, and also by adults who consider it relatively non-toxic; unfortunately this is not the case. The first symptoms are those of upper GI tract irritation which can be severe and haemorrhagic. This can be followed a few hours later by an acute encephalopathy and hepatic necrosis.
Start treatment as soon as possible with
- desferrioxamine 2 g i.m. in 10 ml of water for injection
- washout stomach then leave 5–10 g of desferrioxamine in 100 ml of water in the stomach.

Take blood for
- serum iron
- FBC
- U+E.

If the clinical features suggest severe poisoning (frequent vomiting, bloody diarrhoea or confusion) or the serum iron is >90 mol/l, give desferrioxamine 15 mg/kg/hour to a maximum of 80 mg/kg/24 hours by i.v. infusion.

Tricyclic Antidepressants

Tricyclic antidepressants, when taken in overdosage, can produce a variety of neurological signs; they may cause respiratory depression but this is rarely severe enough to require treatment, the pupils may be dilated and unequal, the muscle tone increased with brisk reflexes and extensor plantar responses. Despite the apparently sinister nature of these signs there is no evidence of neurological damage in these patients when the effects of the drug wear off. The most dangerous feature of tricyclics in overdose is cardiac arrhythmias which are potentially fatal. Conventional anti-arrhythmic treatment can be used although the use of pyridostigmine 1 mg i.m. or i.v., repeated after 15 min if ineffective, has been suggested.

Opiate Overdose

This may occur deliberately, accidentally during drug abuse, or iatrogenically in patients who are sensitive to the respiratory depressant effects of opiates, particularly those with chronic lung disease. The clinical features include depressed conscious level, hypoventilation and pin point pupils.

Naloxone is a specific antidote and the dose is 400 μg i.v. repeated up to three times if the response is poor. The effect of the naloxone is shorter than that of many of the drugs it is used to reverse and may need to be repeated as the effect wears off.

Paraquat Poisoning

Paraquat is extremely toxic, especially when taken in concentrated form. The early effects include painful irritation (and later ulcer-ation) of mucus membranes of the lips, mouth, fauces and eyes where they have come into contact with the paraquat. Later effects include convulsions, increasing dyspnoea due to proliferative alveolitis and bronchiolitis, and renal failure also frequently occurs. There is no specific treatment once the paraquat has been absorbed so the whole aim of treatment is to prevent absorption. This involves careful gastric lavage, firstly because it is important to remove as much of the paraquat as possible and secondly because the ulcerative properties of paraquat make the oesophagus more liable to rupture. A suspension of 150 g of Fuller's earth and 25 g of magnesium sulphate in 500 ml of water should be left in the stomach, and repeated a few hours later. If respiratory problems develop, avoid the use of oxygen if possible as this increases the lung damage.

Solvent Abuse

This is increasingly common particularly among adolescent males. Glues, petrol and organic solvents are most frequently used. The effects differ with individual substances but the overall effects are similar. The acute effects include euphoria, excitement and ataxia and may lead to respiratory depression and coma. The chronic effects are lethargy, anorexia and later renal, hepatic and neurological damage. Any young patient who is admitted to the casualty department with an altered mental state or with depression of conscious level should be examined closely for signs of glue or solvent stains on his clothing and signs of irritation of the eyes and mouth.

SUGGESTED READING

1. H. Matthew, A.A.H. Lawson
    Treatment of Common Acute Poisonings 3rd Ed. 1975
    Edinburgh: Churchill Livingstone

2. J.A. Vale, T.J. Meredith
    Poisoning Diagnosis and Treatment 1st Ed. 1981
    Update Publications

12

MISCELLANEOUS

Management of Anaphylaxis

PREVENTION

Before prescribing any drugs, particularly penicillin, serum products or contrast media, check with the patient, the notes and any warning discs (Medic Alert etc.) for a history of previous allergic reactions.

Emergency drugs such as adrenaline, corticosteriods and antihistamines should be readily available in any areas where drugs are administered.

Treatment of severe anaphylactic reactions:

- check patency of airway.
- assess cardiovascular status, if carotid pulses absent start cardiac massage.
- assess adequacy of respiration.
- give adrenaline 0.5 ml of 1:1000 solution subcutaneously.
- give chlorpheniramine 10 mg i.v.
- give hydrocortisone 200 mg i.v.
- give aminophylline 250 mg by slow i.v. injection if bronchospasm present.
- oxygen in high concentration (35%+).
- give i.v. infusion of N.saline and plasma expander if hypotensive.

Blood Transfusion Reactions

1. Mild reactions include:
   - slight pyrexia

  – flushing
  – itching.
Management
  – slow down rate of transfusion.
  – give an antihistamine (chlorpheniramine 10 mg i.v. or equivalent).
  – monitor pulse, BP and temperature frequently (every 15 min).

2. Severe reactions include the following;
      – urticaria
      – marked pyrexia
      – rigors
      – wheezing
      – hypotension.
Management
  – stop transfusion and send blood back to the lab to be checked.
  – give an antihistamine (chlorpheniramine 10 mg i.v. stat).
  – give hydrocortisone 200 mg i.v. stat.
  – if the reaction includes wheezing or hypotension give adrenaline 0.5 ml of 1:1000 solution subcutaneously.

3. Fluid Overload.
    Patients with severe anaemia or poor cardiac reserve may develop pulmonary oedema during transfusion. To avoid this
      – use packed cells whenever possible, except where the transfusion is given to correct hypotension or hypovolaemia.
      – give a diuretic in the high risk groups (severe anaemia, cardiac insufficiency). Frusemide 20 mg i.v. with each unit of blood is normally adequate.
      – in severe anaemia do not attempt to correct the anaemia completely, at least in one transfusion. Raising the haemoglobin from 4 to 6–7 g/dl should produce symptomatic improvement whereas there is a risk of volume overload in correcting the Hb to 12 g/dl by giving 8–10 units.

Alcohol Toxicity and Withdrawal States

Alcohol-induced medical problems are common, an estimated 5% of medical admissions being due to alcohol related problems. These can take many forms and include:

GIT –liver disease, pancreatitis, increased incidence of peptic ulceration

CNS –delirium tremens, Wernicke's encephalopathy, peripheral neuropathy and myopathy, cerebellar degeneration.

CVS –cardiomyopathy, arrhythmias.

General –increased risk of trauma, aspiration pneumonia, alcohol-induced Cushings syndrome.

ALCOHOL WITHDRAWAL STATES

Mild alcohol withdrawal states are not uncommon in patients who are admitted to hospital for other reasons. Be wary of the patient who becomes restless and slightly confused some time after admission or post-operatively. The full-blown picture of delirium tremens, which includes tremulousness, ataxia, fear, and hallucinations (tactile and visual) is rare, but is a serious condition and may be fatal.

Management
1. If possible have the patient transferred to a side-ward with the lights kept on and as little disturbance as possible, as the patient may interpret sounds, shadows and actions as being threatening.

2. Give chlormethiazole 1–2 g orally 4 hourly
    or chlordiazepoxide 25–50 mg 4 hourly.

3. If oral medication becomes impossible use a chlormethiazole infusion (0.8%) intravenously until the patient is sufficiently sedated (usually requires 40–100 ml of the infusion over 5–10 min)

4. Give high potency B vitamin preparations (parentrovite) 10 ml i.v. daily.

5. Look for a precipitating cause eg. chest infection.

WERNICKE'S ENCEPHALOPATHY

The diagnosis is suggested by the combination of ataxia, nystagmus, disorientation and confabulation. It is due to a deficiency of thiamine and will respond, in some cases completely , to thiamine 50–100 mg daily given parenterally.

"Sections" and Psychiatric Patients

Sections of the 1959 Mental Health Act allow compulsory admission to hospital, detention and treatment.

SECTION 25

This relates to the admission for observation for a period of 28 days. It applies to patients suffering from mental disorder of a nature or degree warranting detention for observation with or without treatment,or to a patient who requires detention for his own health and safety or for the protection of other people.

Two medical recommendations are required: one from an approved medical practitioner and the second from a medical practitioner with previous acquaintance with the patient.

SECTION 29

Admission to hospital for observation in an emergency for not more than 72 hours. One applicant may be a social worker or a relative and only one medical recommendation is needed.

SECTION 30

This concerns the detention of a patient already in hospital, where it seems that a voluntary patient should be detained under the Mental Health Act. The patient may be detained in hospital for 3 days. This requires the recommendation of the consultant.

Of the sections available, the only one in which a hospital doctor is likely to be involved is section 30.

Hypothermia

Hypothermia is defined as a core temperature (for practical purposes normally a rectal temperature) of less than 35°C. Always use a special low reading thermometer when hypothermia is suspected, as normal thermometers only read down to 33°C.

Hypothermia may occur as a primary condition or secondary to any of the causes of coma.

URGENT INVESTIGATIONS

- U+E, blood glucose
- ECG (may show sinus bradycardia, J waves, muscle tremor, prolonged QT, AF)
- blood gases
- drug screen.

MANAGEMENT

Monitor
- rectal temperature continuously or 1/2 hourly
- cardiac rhythm
- respiration
- blood pressure.

TREATMENT

- as for any patient in coma (see "Coma"). Plus
- warm the patient slowly (1°C/hour), using "space" blankets and ordinary blankets.
- treat hypotension with plasma expanders (warm all i.v. fluids).
- give hydrocortisone 200 mg i.v. q.d.s until recovered.
- treat cardiac arrhythmias as they arise; ventricular fibrillation is not uncommon in severe hypothermia (see "Cardiac Arrest").
- infection, particularly chest infection, is common.

Malaria

In *Plasmodium vivax*, *P.ovale*, and *P.malariae* infections the clinical features are seldom severe, and are limited to rigors, fever and sweating, with <1% of red cells being parasitised.
Falciparum malaria ranges from mild to fatal; the clinical features include
Cerebral – headache, drowsiness, confusion, convulsions, coma.
GI and liver – abdominal pain, diarrhoea, hepatocellular jaundice.
Pulmonary – adult respiratory distress syndrome, pulmonary oedema (fluid overload)
Renal – acute tubular necrosis, immune complex nephritis, nephrotic syndrome, renal cortical necrosis.
Haematological – anaemia, coagulation defects, DIC.

INVESTIGATIONS

"Thick" blood film – in light parasitaemia several films may have to be examined before malarial parasites are seen.
FBC – anaemia, haemolysis, DIC.
U+E – renal impairment.
LFTs – elevated bilirubin.
chest X-ray – pulmonary oedema, adult respiratory distress

syndrome.
urine – protein, haemoglobinuria.

TREATMENT

Drugs
Plasmodium vivax, ovale, malariae and uncomplicated *falciparum* in chloroquine sensitive areas;
Chloroquine
  – 600 mg oral stat
  – 300 mg 6 hours later
  – 300 mg daily for 2 days
Severe falciparum malaria
  – quinine dihydrochloride 5–10 mg/kg (max. 500 mg) by i.v. infusion 12 hourly until oral treatment is possible.
  – oral chloroquine regime as above.
or – in chloroquine resistant areas quinine sulphate 600 mg 12 hourly for 3 days then Fansidar 3 tablets stat.

NOTE
Reduce the dose of antimalarial drugs if there is evidence of severe liver impairment.

General Supportive Treatment of Complicated Falciparum Malaria
  – avoid fluid overload (patients may appear clinically dehydrated due to fever but in fact are not).
  – treat pulmonary oedema if present.
  – if severely anaemic (Hb<6 g/dl)transfuse with care, giving not more than 2 units of blood in 24 hours.
  – treat convulsions with diazepam
  – do NOT attempt to treat DIC with anticoagulants.

Malaria Prophylaxis
  – Commence 1 week before going and continue for 4 weeks after return.
  Chloroquine sensitive areas
  – proguanil 100–200 mg daily
or – pyrimethamine 25 mg weekly.
  Chloroquine resistant areas
  – Maloprim (pyrimethamine 12.5 mg plus dapsone 100 mg) 1 tablet weekly

−Fansidar (pyrimethamine 25 mg plus sulfadoxime 500 mg weekly) 1 tablet weekly.

Pyrexia of Unknown Origin

DEFINITION

A pyrexial illness unexplained after a history and examination

CAUSES

- TB.
- infective endocarditis.
- abscess: intra-abdominal, hepatic, biliary, renal.
- other infections including:

bacterial – brucella, typhoid, paratyphoid, meningococcaemia, syphilis.

viral – cytomegalovirus, infectious mononucleosis

protozoal – malaria, amoebiasis, toxoplasmosis.

rickettsial – Q fever, psittacosis, mycoplasma.

- neoplasia: Hodgkin's lymphoma, non-Hodgkin's lymphoma, hypernephroma, leukaemia, hepatoma, atrial myxoma.
- collagen vascular disease.
- drugs: methyl dopa, phenytoin, salicylates, isoniazid.
- other causes: sarcoid, inflammatory bowel disease, Whipple's disease, Familial Mediterranean Fever, Weber Christian disease, hypothalamic lesions, thyroiditis, phaeochromocytoma.

HISTORY

Pay particular attention to
- exposure to infections
- contact with animals
- travel
- occupational hazards
- prior surgery or trauma
- drugs.

It is important to keep the history and physical examination continually under review, and frequently useful for someone previously unconnected with the case to repeat the history and examination without prior knowledge of the situation.

INVESTIGATIONS

Initial Screen
- FBC, differential WBC, and ESR
- blood film
- U+E, LFTs
- blood cultures (6)
- sera to store for future studies (eg paired sera for serology)
- serum immunoglobulins
- ANF, RW
- chest X-ray, plain abdominal X-ray
- urine for blood, protein and culture
- sputum culture.

Other Tests
Futher investigations at this stage depend on clues from the history and examination and the results of the initial investigations, and may include some of the following:

Serology – viral titres, Paul-Bunnel or Monospot, brucella titres, enteric fever, syphilis, toxoplasma dye test, amoebic fluorescent antibody test, coxiella antibodies, Felix-Weil reaction (rickettsia), chlamydia antibodies (psittacosis).

Ultrasound – very useful for intra-abdominal lesions.

Isotope scans – liver scan
          – gallium scan (taken up by inflammatory or neoplastic lesions).

Computerised axial tomography

Radiology – IVP
          – lymphangiography.

Management of Near Drowning

IMMEDIATE PROBLEMS

Is cardiopulmonary resuscitation needed?
(see under "Cardiac Arrest").

Is ventilation adequate? If not, procede to intubation and artificial ventilation.

URGENT INVESTIGATIONS

- blood gases
- electrolytes
- chest X-ray, look for pulmonary oedema
- FBC

NEXT STEPS

1. Monitor ventilation
   - give oxygen by mask.
   - aim to keep pO_2 > 8.0 kPa (60 mmHg).
   - pulmonary oedema is common after inhalation of water.
   - if the patient deteriorates, proceed to artificial ventilation.

2. Measure temperature with a low-reading rectal thermometer as hypothermia is common.

3. Put up an i.v. infusion
   - give 5% dextrose in sea-water drowning.
   - give normal saline in fresh-water drowning.
   - give bicarbonate to keep pH above 7.2.
   - give plasma to expand the circulation as necessary.
   - electrolyte abnormalities occasionally need specific treatment.
   - warm all i.v. fluids.

4. High dose steroids are often advised though no benefit is proven e.g. hydrocortisone 500 mg i.v. 6 hourly.

5. Give i.v. broad spectrum antibiotics. Watch for signs of chest infection or lung abscess, especially when immersion was in polluted water.
   Culture sputum and check for unusual organisms.

NOTE

   - in the event of a cardiac arrest, do not give up too soon as low body temperature means that recovery is possible after a longer period of asystole or apnoea than usual.

– monitor chest X-ray in recovery period, looking for respiratory complications.

– haemolysis is sometimes seen in freshwater drowning but rarely needs treatment.

"Drug Rashes"

URTICARIA

– pink raised wheal with pale centre, due to histamine release, associated with anaphylaxis.

– penicillins, barbiturates, aspirin, contrast media.

TOXIC ERYTHEMA

– is the commonest reaction, and is a measles-like rash deep red to bluish in colour.

– ampicillin, phenylbutazone, phenothiazines, co-trimoxazole, thiazides, sulphonylureas.

ERYTHEMA MULTIFORME

– fixed urticated target lesions, may be haemorrhagic or blistered; severe cases (Stevens-Johnson syndrome) include gross blistering, erosion of the mucous membranes and systemic features including fever and arthralgia:

– sulphonamides, phenylbutazone, dichlorphenazone, diflunisal, barbiturates.

ALLERGIC VASCULITIS

– involvement of deep vessels leads to erythema nodosum, and involvement of superficial vessels to fixed dark red lesions, blood blisters and necrotic ulceration of the skin.

– methyl dopa, thiazides, phenylbutazone, phenytoin.

PURPURA

– rust coloured petechial rash over ankles, thighs and buttocks particularly.

– phenobarbitone, meprobamate, carbromal.

FIXED DRUG REACTIONS

- annular patches of erythema which swell and itch
- quinine, dapsone, phenolphthalein, chlordiazepoxide, tetracyclines.

HYPERPIGMENTATION

- chlorpromazine, oral contraceptive pill.

PHOTOSENSITIVTY

- exposed skin may blister.
- demeclocycline, phenothiazines, nalidixic acid, sulphonamides, thiazides, sulphonylureas.

LUPUS ERYTHEMATOSUS

- hydralazine, procainamide, phenytoin.

LICHEN PLANUS

- violaceous, intensely itchy papules, mouth ulceration frequently present.
- gold, methyl dopa.

Glossary

ACTH	– adrenocorticotrophic hormone
ADH	– anti-diuretic hormone
AF	– atrial fibrillation
AFBs	– acid fast bacilli
AIR	– accelerated idioventricular rhythm
ANF	– anti-nuclear factor
APTT	– accelerated partial thromboplastin time
B^1	– thiamine
B^6	– pyridoxine
B^{12}	– cyanocobalamin
BCG	– Bacille Calmette Guerin
CAT	– computerised axial tomography
CFT	– complement fixation test
CHB	– complete heart block
CLL	– chronic lymphatic leukaemia
CML	– chronic myeloid leukaemia
CVP	– central venous pressure
DC	– direct current
DIC	– disseminated intravascular coagulation
DVT	– deep vein thrombosis
ECG	– electrocardiogram
EEG	– electroencephalogram
ESR	– erythrocyte sedimentation rate
ET	– endotracheal tube
FEV	– forced expiratory volume
FTI	– free thyroxine index
FVC	– forced vital capacity
G6PD	– glucose-6-phosphate dehydrogenase deficiency
GGT	– gamma glutamyl transferase
GTN	– glyceryl trinitrate
GTT	– glucose tolerance test

IPPV	–	intermittent positive pressure ventilation
ITP	–	idiopathic thrombocytopaenic purpura
IVP	–	intravenous pyelogram
JVP	–	jugular venous pressure
LAHB	–	left anterior hemiblock
LDH	–	lactic dehydrogenase
LP	–	lumbar puncture
LPHB	–	left posterior hemiblock
MS	–	Multiple sclerosis
MSU	–	mid stream urine
NAP	–	neutrophil alkaline phosphatase
NSAID	–	non steroidal anti-inflammatory drugs
PA	–	pulmonary artery, postero-anterior
PE	–	pulmonary embolism
PRV	–	polycythaemia rubra vera
PT	–	prothrombin time
PTH·	–	parathyroid hormone
RA	–	rheumatoid arthritis, right atrium
RBBB	–	right bundle branch block
RBC	–	red blood cell
RV	–	right ventricle, residual volume
RW	–	Rose Waaler
SBE	–	sub-acute bacterial endocarditis
SLE	–	systemic lupus erythematosus
SVT	–	supra ventricular tachycardia
TIA	–	transient ischaemic attack
TIP	–	terminal interphalangeal joint
T	–	tri-iodothyronine
T4	–	thyroxine
TB	–	tuberculosis
TBG	–	thyroid binding globulin
TLC	–	total lung capacity
TRH	–	thyrotrophin releasing hormone
TSH	–	thyroid stimulating hormone
U+E	–	urea and electrolytes
VDRL	–	venereal disease reference laboratory test
VF	–	ventricular fibrillation
VSD	–	ventricular septal defect
VT	–	ventricular tachycardia
WR	–	Wasserman reaction
ZN	–	Ziehl-Neelson stain

INDEX